NUTRITION
AND
DENTAL HEALTH

NUTRITION AND DENTAL HEALTH

SECOND EDITION

Ann Ehrlich, C.D.A., M.A.

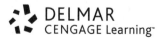
DELMAR
CENGAGE Learning™

Australia • Brazil • Japan • Korea • Mexico • Singapore • Spain • United Kingdom • United States

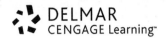
DELMAR
CENGAGE Learning™

**Nutrition and Dental Health,
Second Edition**
Ann Ehrlich

Publisher: David C. Gordon

Acquisitions Editor: Adrianne C. Williams

Manager, Art, Design, and Production:
Russell Schneck

Production Coordinator: Jennifer Gaines

Cover Design: Timothy J. Conners

For product information and technology assistance, contact us at
Cengage Learning Customer & Sales Support, 1-800-354-9706

For permission to use material from this text or product,
submit all requests online at **www.cengage.com/permissions**
Further permissions questions can be emailed to
permissionrequest@cengage.com

Library of Congress Control Number: 93-43043

ISBN-13: 978-0-8273-5716-7

ISBN-10: 0-8273-5716-8

Delmar
Executive Woods
5 Maxwell Drive
Clifton Park, NY 12065
USA

Cengage Learning is a leading provider of customized learning solutions with office locations around the globe, including Singapore, the United Kingdom, Australia, Mexico, Brazil, and Japan. Locate your local office at
www.cengage.com/global

Cengage Learning products are represented in Canada by
Nelson Education, Ltd.

To learn more about Delmar, visit **www.cengage.com/delmar**

Purchase any of our products at your local bookstore or at our preferred online store **www.cengagebrain.com**

Printed in the United States of America
12 13 14 15 16   22 21 20 19 18

CONTENTS _____

PREFACE   **ix**

CHAPTER **1**   **INTRODUCTION TO NUTRITION**
               AND DENTAL HEALTH   **1**

               Objectives   **1**
               Nutrition and Dental Health   **2**
               How This Book Is Organized   **4**
               What Is Nutrition?   **5**
               Nutrition Theories   **6**
               Health   **7**
               Review Exercises   **8**

CHAPTER **2**   **DIGESTION, ABSORPTION,**
               AND METABOLISM   **11**

               Objectives   **11**
               Overview of Digestion   **12**
               Digestive Changes in the Mouth   **16**
               Digestive Changes in the Stomach   **17**
               Digestive Changes in the Small Intestine   **18**
               Functions of the Large Intestine   **19**
               Absorption   **20**
               Metabolism   **21**
               Review Exercises   **23**

CHAPTER **3**   **KEY NUTRIENTS**   **26**

               Objectives   **26**
               Key Nutrients   **27**

Nutrients Work Individually and
Together   28
Nutrient Needs   29
Nutrients and Supplements   31
Energy Needs   34
Review Exercises   37

CHAPTER **4**   **CARBOHYDRATES**   40

Objectives   40
Major Functions of Carbohydrates   41
Sources of Carbohydrates   42
Classification of Carbohydrates   42
Glucose and Glycogen   45
More About Sugars   46
Dietary Fiber   49
Review Exercises   54

CHAPTER **5**   **PROTEINS, FATS, AND
WATER**   57

Objectives   57
Proteins   58
Fats   62
Water   66
Review Exercises   68

CHAPTER **6**   **VITAMINS**   71

Objectives   71
The Functions of Vitamins   72
Daily Vitamin Needs   73
Fat-Soluble Vitamins   74
Water-Soluble Vitamins   78
Review Exercises   87

CHAPTER **7** **MINERALS, TRACE ELEMENTS, AND ELECTROLYTES**   **90**

Objectives   **90**
The Functions of Minerals   **91**
Minerals   **93**
Trace Elements   **101**
Electrolytes   **105**
Review Exercises   **108**

CHAPTER **8** **DIETARY GUIDELINES**   **111**

Objectives   **111**
Overview   **112**
Dietary Guidelines for Americans   **112**
The *Food Guide Pyramid*   **117**
Food Labeling Information   **123**
Diet Diary   **125**
Review Exercises   **127**

CHAPTER **9** **SPECIAL NUTRITIONAL NEEDS**   **131**

Objectives   **131**
Overview of Special Needs   **132**
Prenatal and Pregnancy Needs   **132**
Infancy   **133**
The Preschool Child   **135**
The School-Age Child   **136**
Adolescence   **137**
Adulthood   **140**
The Elderly   **143**
Review Exercises   **149**

CHAPTER **10** **SPECIAL DIETS FOR DENTAL PATIENTS**   **152**

Objectives   **152**
Introduction to Special Diets   **153**

Types of Special Diets   154
Modified Diets   158
Review Exercises   165

CHAPTER **11** **THE ROLE OF FLUORIDES IN
                PREVENTIVE DENTISTRY**   167

Objectives   167
Overview of Fluorides   168
Systemic Fluorides   171
Topical Fluorides   175
Review Exercises   178

CHAPTER **12** **THE ROLE OF PLAQUE
                CONTROL IN PREVENTIVE
                DENTISTRY**   181

Objectives   181
Dental Plaque   182
Food and Dental Plaque   184
Personal Oral Hygiene (POH)   187
Review Exercises   199

APPENDIX A   **ANSWER KEYS**   202

APPENDIX B   **CROSSWORD PUZZLES AND
                ANSWER KEYS**   206

                GLOSSARY   210

                REFERENCES   231

                INDEX   235

PREFACE

Many exciting changes have come about since the first edition of **Nutrition and Dental Health** was published in 1987. These changes are so extensive that, instead of merely revising an existing text, the entire book has been rewritten.

This second edition reflects exciting research findings that ongoing supplies of fluorides can help to remineralize and repair teeth damaged by acid attacks from dental plaque. These findings place the preventive dentistry emphasis on the need to provide fluorides and, of course, on the need for regular plaque removal.

In keeping with the tradition of the first edition, the first part of the book is devoted to a simplified explanation of nutrition and how the reader may apply this knowledge in his or her daily life. There are updates here too with the inclusion of the Food Pyramid, changing guidelines, and new information about how the foods we eat impact our health now and as we age.

The book is divided into twelve chapters. There are ten exercises and a suggested class activity at the end of each chapter. The answer keys for the exercises are found in **Appendix A**.

After the chapters, there is a glossary containing more than 175 terms that are found in the text. **Appendix B** consists of two crossword puzzles and their solutions. These puzzles are based on the terms found in the glossary.

It is my hope that you will enjoy this study of nutrition and preventive dentistry, and that you will apply it to enhance your professional work and to improve the quality of life for yourself and your family.

I wish to thank the Delmar Staff for their assistance and guidance in this project. I also greatly appreciate the valuable input from the following reviewers who helped to make this a better text.

Betty Ladley Finkbeiner, CDA, RDA, BS, MS
Department Chairperson
Dental Assistant Program
Washtenaw Community College
Ann Arbor, MI

Paulette Yelton, CDA, MPA
Assistant Professor
Dental Assistant Program
East Tennessee State University
Elizabethton, TN

Mary K. Smith, RDH
Niskayuna, NY

Eugenia Bearden, RDH, ME
Assistant Professor of Dental Hygiene
Dental Hygiene Department
Clayton State College
Morrow, GA

Lori A. Burch, RDA
Dental Department
ConCorde Career Institute
North Hollywood, CA

Dianne McCarley, RDA, CDA
Adult Educator
National Education Centers
Irvine, CA

CHAPTER 1

INTRODUCTION TO NUTRITION AND DENTAL HEALTH

OBJECTIVES _____

After studying this chapter, you should be able to:

- list and describe the three major factors that influence nutrition and dental health.
- describe what is meant by the terms diet and adequate diet.
- differentiate between the terms diet and nutrition.
- define malnutrition, undernutrition, and overnutrition.

NUTRITION AND DENTAL HEALTH

Nutrition and dental health are not separate topics; you must have one in order to have the other. Being well-nourished throughout life is essential for the development and maintenance of sound teeth and tissues. On the other hand, if the individual does not have sound teeth and a healthy mouth he cannot eat properly and may suffer from nutritional disorders.

Preventive Dentistry

Three forces must be present for dental decay to occur (Fig. 1-1). These are: (1) an unprotected tooth, (2) bacteria in dental plaque, and (3) an energy source for the bacteria. The bacteria in the plaque uses its food source (sugars in the mouth) to create acid which attacks the enamel of the teeth.

Preventive dentistry has long recognized that if any one of these three factors is removed dental decay will be prevented. Formerly the role of nutrition in achieving dental health consisted of the traditional "*avoid sweets, and see your dentist twice a year.*" Today we recognize that effective preventive dentistry must include the role of general nutrition, fluorides, and plaque control.

General Nutrition

General nutrition consists of many parts. These include learning:

- how the body utilizes the foods we eat.
- to identify nutritional needs and the food sources that will meet these needs.
- the role of federal guidelines for selecting foods to meet nutritional needs.
- how to apply this knowledge in your own life and how to share this information with others.

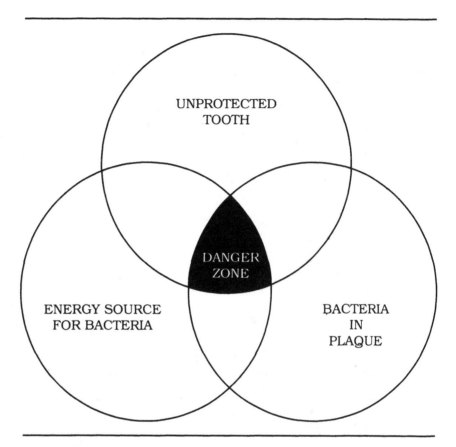

FIGURE 1-1   Three factors which must be present to cause dental decay are: an unprotected tooth, bacteria in plaque, and an energy source for the bacteria.

Fluorides

Fluorides, which are nutrients, play a major role in making teeth more resistant to the **acid attacks** that cause dental decay. Understanding how these benefits are best acquired for each individual plays an important role in preventive dentistry. This is discussed in Chapter 11.

Plaque Control

Dental plaque, which is made up of bacteria, is the major causative factor in tooth decay and periodontal disease. This is discussed in Chapter 12.

Plaque control focuses on two areas. One is modification of the diet to limit the nutrients available for the plaque to use. The second is the thorough removal of all plaque daily through toothbrushing and other oral hygiene measures.

Patients must learn these techniques and be motivated to follow through on them as part of a daily home care program.

HOW THIS BOOK IS ORGANIZED

The primary goal of this book is to help you learn about these three factors and apply them effectively in your own life. A secondary goal is to help you learn to communicate this information to dental patients so they may move toward better dental health.

Toward these goals, information is presented in the following sequence:

1. digestion, or how the body uses the food that is eaten,
2. nutrients,
3. guidelines for selecting a healthy diet—specific needs and special diets for dental patients,
4. the role of fluorides in dental health,
5. teaching plaque control.

WHAT IS NUTRITION?

The term **diet** refers to the food that is taken into the mouth. An **adequate diet** meets all of the nutritional needs of an individual and provides some degree of protection for periods of increased needs such as illness or extreme stress.

The term **nutrition** refers to the manner in which the body utilizes the nutrients contained in foods eaten. **Good nutrition** means that the body is well nourished by having received and put to work foods containing essential nutrients in the amounts needed. A well-nourished person is likely to be healthy, of optimal weight for frame size, and mentally and physically alert.

The term **malnutrition** is used to describe any disorder of nutrition or undesirable health status that is due to either a lack of or an excess of nutrient supply. Although we usually think of malnutrition as undernutrition (lack of nutrients), the definition also includes overnutrition (too much food) which is an equally serious problem.

Undernutrition is an undesirable health status resulting from a lack of healthy nutrients. In the young it may inhibit growth, delay maturation, limit physical activity, and interfere with learning. At all ages it makes the individual more susceptible to diseases.

The major diseases resulting from undernutrition are rarely seen in this country; however, they are a large problem in developing nations where much of the population lacks adequate food.

Overnutrition, which is the intake of excessive nutrients, may lead to obesity and its many related diseases. **Obesity** is an accumulation of excessive fat in the body that results in body weight beyond the limitations of skeletal and physical requirements. In our culture, overnutrition is a far more common and serious problem than is undernutrition (Fig. 1-2).

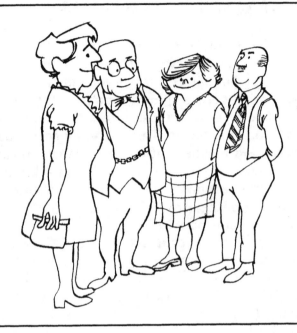

FIGURE 1-2   In the United States, overnutrition is more common than undernutrition.

NUTRITION THEORIES

Everyone should be an expert on the subject of nutrition because our well-being and survival depend upon the food choices we make daily. Although interested and concerned, most of us are also justifiably confused because nutrition is a fascinating but complex and somewhat controversial subject.

We are surrounded by sound information and much misinformation, and it is difficult to tell which is which. There are theories without scientific basis, conflicting views, and self-proclaimed experts who lack professional credentials.

This wealth of misinformation is most obvious in the

area of "weight loss diets." It seems as if each week there is a new "surefire, can't-miss fad diet." The fact that new diets are constantly being developed proves that the old ones don't work.

The information presented in this text does not represent the latest fad. Instead, after extensive research information has been drawn from respected sources. A list of these references is included at the end of the book.

The emphasis throughout the text is to enable you to apply the basic principles of good nutrition in your own life, make informed food choices, and evaluate nutrition information from other sources.

HEALTH

According to the World Health Organization (WHO) definition, **health** is "a state of complete physical, mental, and social well-being and not merely the absence of disease or infirmity."

Good nutrition is vital, but it is only one of the factors contributing to good health. Other key factors include:

- exercise,
- lifestyle,
- stress reduction, and
- preventive care.

These factors are beyond the scope of this book; however, you are encouraged to continue your studies and to learn about them, too.

REVIEW EXERCISES _____

MULTIPLE CHOICE

Circle the correct answer for each question.

1. The term _____ refers to the foods we eat and the way the body uses them.

   a) diet
   b) nutrition
   c) metabolism

2. Fluorides are _____.

   a) nutrients
   b) medications used in preventive dentistry
   c) the major causative factor of periodontal disease

3. The term _____ is used to describe any disorder of nutrition, or undesirable health status, that is due to either a lack of or an excess of nutrient supply.

   a) adequate diet
   b) malnutrition
   c) nourishment

4. The role of nutrition in dental health is limited to helping the patient avoid sweets.

   a) True
   b) false

5. _____ is/are the major causative factor(s) in periodontal disease.

   a) Dental plaque
   b) Excessive sweets
   c) Malnutrition

6. In our culture, _____ is a common and serious nutritional problem.

   a) overnutrition
   b) undernutrition

7. _____ means that the body is well nourished by
having received and put to work essential nutrients
in the amounts needed.

   a) An adequate diet
   b) Good nutrition
   c) Overnutrition

8. _____ is an accumulation of excessive fat in the
body which results in body weight beyond the limitations of skeletal and physical requirements.

   a) Obecity
   b) Obescity
   c) Obesity

9. The term _____ refers to the foods taken into the
mouth.

   a) adequate nutrition
   b) diet
   c) malnutrition

10. _____ is a state of complete physical, mental, and
social well-being.

   a) Adequate diet
   b) Good nutrition
   c) Health

SUGGESTED CLASS ACTIVITY

Collect news items about nutrition. These can be found in newspapers, general interest magazines, health newsletters, etc., or on television. (For television items, note the name of the program, date, and time that it was aired.) In class, be prepared to discuss how you, as a consumer, can determine how accurate these news stories are.

Also look for news items and advertisements concerning weight-loss diets. When reviewing the weight-loss diets and advertisements, note the claims that are made. Again, as a consumer, discuss how you would evaluate the truth of these claims.

CHAPTER 2

DIGESTION, ABSORPTION, AND METABOLISM

OBJECTIVES _____

After studying this chapter, you should be able to:

- differentiate between mechanical and chemical digestion.
- name the enzymes involved in the digestive changes that occur in the mouth, stomach, small intestine, and large intestine.
- state the substance acted upon by each of these enzymes.
- state the site where each type of nutrient is digested and absorbed into the body.
- define metabolism and differentiate between anabolism and catabolism.

OVERVIEW OF DIGESTION

Digestion is the process by which foods are broken down into their nutrients. The major components of the digestive system are shown in Figure 2-1. **Absorption** is the process of taking these nutrients into the circulation so that they can be used by the body. **Metabolism** encompasses the chemical changes that determine the final use of the individual nutrients.

All three of the factors must be present and working effectively in order for the body to utilize the nutrients in the foods which have been selected and eaten. The nutrients which are mentioned in this chapter are explained in greater detail in the chapters that follow.

The digestion process consists of two parts: mechanical digestion and chemical digestion (Table 2-1).

Mechanical Digestion

Mechanical digestion includes the *chewing* of food, the *churning* actions of the stomach, and *peristalsis*, which is the rhythmic contractions of the intestines. These movements break food into smaller and smaller particles and mix the food with the digestive juices. In addition, peristalsis continually moves the food mass through the intestines.

Chemical Digestion

Chemical digestion is the action of enzymes as they break foods down into simpler forms which can then be absorbed by the body. An **enzyme** is a substance that causes a chemical change, or breakdown, in other substances. Enzymes are specific in their action. This means that a particular digestive enzyme will act only on a certain kind of foodstuff and will not produce action on any other. For

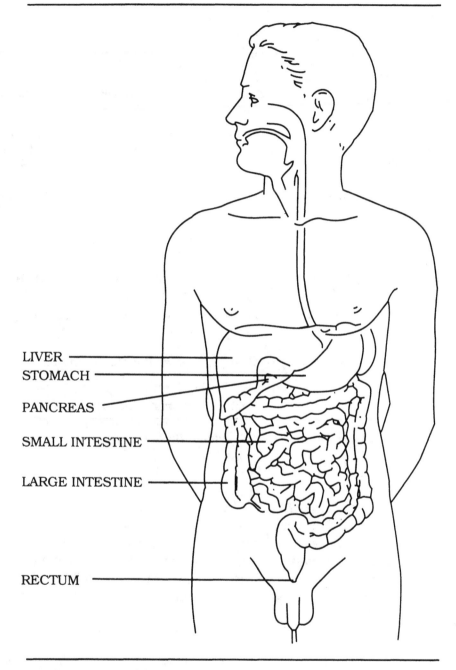

LIVER

STOMACH

PANCREAS

SMALL INTESTINE

LARGE INTESTINE

RECTUM

FIGURE 2-1 Major structures of the digestive system.

Site	Digestive Action
Mouth	Chewing begins the mechanical breakdown of food.
	Beginning chemical breakdown and digestion of carbohydrates. Carbohydrates are the only nutrients "digested" in the mouth.
Stomach	Churning action for mechanical breakdown of food.
	Limited chemical breakdown of proteins and fats.
Small Intestine	Further chemical breakdown of carbohydrates, proteins, and fats.
	Absorption of most nutrients including vitamins and minerals.
Large Intestine	Absorption of additional vitamins.
	Absorption of water.
	Discharge of waste materials.

TABLE 2-1 Sites of Digestive Action

example, an enzyme that digests fat will not digest starch. Table 2-2 summarizes enzyme activity in digestion.

Many of these enzymes require additional substances known as **coenzymes,** which are produced by the body from some of the vitamins and minerals which have been ingested. (**Ingested** means eaten or taken into the body.)

Location	Enzyme	Acts Upon
Mouth	Salivary amylase	Carbohydrates
Gastric juice in stomach	Protease	Proteins
Gastric juice in stomach	Rennin	Milk casein
Gastric juice in stomach	Lipase	Emulsified fats
Pancreatic juice in small intestine	Trypsin	Proteins
Pancreatic juice in small intestine	Lipase	Fats
Pancreatic juice in small intestine	Amylase	Starch
Intestinal juice in small intestine	Peptidases	Proteins
Intestinal juice in small intestine	Sucrase	Sucrose
Intestinal juice in small intestine	Maltase	Maltose
Intestinal juice in small intestine	Lactase	Lactose

TABLE 2-2 Digestive Enzymes

DIGESTIVE CHANGES IN THE MOUTH

Mechanical Digestion

The first change in food is the mechanical action that occurs during chewing. Chewing, which is also known as **mastication,** breaks the food into small pieces and mixes it with saliva. The process of mixing food with saliva is known as **insalivation.**

Chemical Digestion

Salivary amylase is the enzyme found in saliva. It acts only on carbohydrates. It begins the process of breaking complex carbohydrates down into simpler sugars which the body can use.

The Special Role of Saliva

In addition to aiding in digestion, an adequate supply of saliva is necessary to help protect the teeth in three important ways:

1. The saliva constantly flushes the mouth to clear food debris that may act as a food supply for the bacteria in plaque.
2. It reduces the pH (acidity) of the waste products produced by plaque. This helps to limit the damage caused by these acid attacks. (Acid attacks are explained in Chapter 12.)
3. Saliva is the source of systemic fluorides and minerals needed for the remineralization of the damaged dental enamel. (This process is explained in Chapter 11.)

When there is not an adequate supply of saliva because of illness, drugs, or radiation therapy, the decay rate increases rapidly.

DIGESTIVE CHANGES IN THE STOMACH

The stomach serves as a temporary storehouse for food. It also brings about partial digestion of protein and prepares food for further digestion in the small intestine.

Mechanical and Chemical Digestion

In the stomach, food is continually churned and mixed with gastric juice until it reaches a liquid consistency known as **chyme. Gastric juice** contains hydrochloric acid, the enzymes protease, rennin, and lipase, and other substances.

Hydrochloric acid serves four important functions:

1. It swells the proteins so they can be more easily attacked by the enzymes.
2. It provides the acid medium necessary for the action of pepsin.
3. It increases the solubility of calcium and iron salts so that they are absorbed more readily.
4. It reduces the activity of harmful bacteria that may have been present in the food.

The enzyme **pepsin** acts upon proteins by splitting them into smaller molecules. The enzyme **rennin** acts on casein (one of the proteins in milk) and breaks it down into calcium caseinate.

The enzyme **lipase** has some effect on emulsified fats such as those found in cream and egg yolk. It begins the process of changing them into fatty acids and glycerol. However, most of the digestion of fats takes place in the small intestine. Very little digestion of carbohydrates and other fats occurs in the stomach.

Food remains in the stomach for varying lengths of time, depending on the type of food. Carbohydrates leave the stomach very quickly. Protein leaves more quickly than fat. Smaller amounts of food leave the stomach in less time than a large meal.

DIGESTIVE CHANGES IN THE SMALL INTESTINE

Chemical Digestion

Most digestive activity takes place in the small intestine through the combined actions of **bile, pancreatic juice,** and **intestinal juice.**

Bile

Bile is essential for fat digestion. It is manufactured by the liver, stored in the gallbladder, and released directly into the small intestine.

Bile breaks fats down into tiny globules, allowing the fat-splitting enzymes to have greater contact with the fat molecules. This process of breaking down fat is known as **emulsification.**

Pancreatic Juice

Pancreatic juice, which is secreted by the pancreas, is also released directly into the small intestine. Pancreatic juice contains these enzymes:

- **Trypsin** which acts on protein by breaking it down into even smaller molecules and some amino acids.
- **Lipase** which completes the digestion of fats.
- **Amylase** which breaks starch down into maltose.

Intestinal Juice

Intestinal juice, which is produced in the intestine, contains additional protein and sugar-splitting enzymes.

- **Peptidases** complete the breakdown of proteins into amino acids.
- **Sucrase** brings about the change of sucrose into glucose and fructose.
- **Maltase** acts on the maltose molecule to yield glucose.
- **Lactase** breaks lactose into the simple sugars glucose and galactose.

FUNCTIONS OF THE LARGE INTESTINE

Digestion has been essentially completed by the time the food mass reaches the large intestine. Here bacteria synthesize vitamin K and some of the vitamins of the B-complex group. These and electrolytes (principally sodium) are absorbed from the large intestine.

Water is absorbed here also, and gradually the intestinal contents take on a solid consistency. These solid wastes are eliminated through the rectum as **feces.** The feces contain fibers of food, small amounts of undigested food, bile salts, cholesterol, mucus, bacteria, and broken-down cellular wastes.

Also eliminated are 20 to 70 percent of ingested calcium, 80 to 85 percent of ingested iron, and considerable amounts of phosphates.

Elimination

Solid waste is excreted from the large intestine through the rectum. The frequency of elimination of the feces, commonly referred to as a bowel movement, varies considerably from individual to individual.

One person's bowels can move as frequently as three times a day and another's as infrequently as three times a week, and in both cases be perfectly normal.

Constipation is defined as the infrequent or difficult evacuation of feces. Many people believe that constipation, or irregularity, is the failure to evacuate the bowel daily. This belief is not accurate. The key to regularity is the normal bowel frequency for the individual.

ABSORPTION

After digestion of the nutrients is complete, the simplified end products are ready to be absorbed. No absorption of nutrients takes place in the mouth or stomach, although water is absorbed to some extent.

Most nutrients are absorbed through the small intestine. These include monosaccharides from carbohydrates such as glucose, fructose, and galactose; fatty acids and glycerides from fats; and amino acids from proteins. Vitamins and minerals liberated in the process of digestion are also absorbed.

When absorption is impaired, the body cannot properly utilize the nutrients that were eaten.

METABOLISM

The various absorbed nutrient components are carried to the cells as ready-to-use materials to produce the substances needed by the body to sustain life. Such substances fill two essential needs.

First, they produce energy required by the body. Second, they maintain a balance between the building up and breaking down of tissue. The terms **homeostasis** and **dynamic equilibrium** are used to describe this balance.

Metabolism is an inclusive term that describes all the changes that take place in the body. Essentially, it means those processes that are concerned with the use of the nutrients absorbed into the blood following digestion.

The **metabolic rate** is the speed and efficiency with which the body converts food into useful nutrients. Here the term efficiency means how much energy the body requires for this conversion process.

Anabolism and Catabolism

The two phases of metabolism are **anabolism** (the construction phase) and **catabolism** (the destruction phase).

Anabolism is concerned with the conversion of the simple compounds derived from nutrients into substances that the body cells can use. An example of anabolism is the formation of new body tissues.

Catabolism involves the breaking down of body tissues. An example of catabolism is in the breakdown of tissue associated with surgery, burns, and other trauma. (**Trauma** means injury or wound.)

The term catabolism also refers to the process whereby substances are converted into simpler compounds which release the energy necessary for the proper functioning of the body cells.

REVIEW EXERCISES _____

MULTIPLE CHOICE

Circle the correct answer for each question.

1. Salivary amylase is an enzyme that acts on _____.

    a) carbohydrates
    b) fats
    c) protein

2. Most nutrients are absorbed from the _____.

    a) large intestine
    b) small intestine
    c) stomach

3. A/An _____ is a substance that causes a chemical change in other substances.

    a) catabolism
    b) chyme
    c) enzyme

4. The movement of the intestines which mixes food with digestive juices is called _____.

    a) insalivation
    b) mastication
    c) peristalsis

5. The enzyme lactase is found in _____.

    a) bile
    b) intestinal juice
    c) pancreatic juice

6. The term _____ describes the speed and efficiency with which the body converts food into useful nutrients.

   a) absorption
   b) digestion
   c) metabolic rate

7. The breaking down of body tissue after an injury such as a burn is an example of _____.

   a) anabolism
   b) catabolism
   c) metabolism

8. Hydrochloric acid is found in _____ juice.

   a) gastric
   b) intestinal
   c) pancreatic

9. The churning action of the stomach is a form of _____.

   a) insalivation
   b) mechanical digestion
   c) peristalsis

10. _____ is the process by which foods are broken down into their nutrients.

   a) Anabolism
   b) Digestion
   c) Metabolism

SUGGESTED CLASS ACTIVITY

Make a list or collect examples of advertisements you see for "digestive aids." These could be on television, in magazines and newspapers, or on products you have seen in stores.

Each of these products is promoted as *the solution to a problem*," and most will probably be for indigestion or constipation. However, there are also many other types of products so try to collect examples of as many different types as possible.

In class, be prepared to discuss the types of problems that products are supposed to solve. Then discuss how these problems affect an individual's general nutrition and good health.

CHAPTER 3

KEY NUTRIENTS

OBJECTIVES _____

After studying this chapter, you should be able to:

- define the term nutrients and describe the role they play in maintaining health.
- discuss how nutrients work individually and together.
- define Recommended Dietary Allowances (RDAs), United States Recommended Daily Allowances (U.S. RDAs), estimated safe and adequate daily dietary intake (ESIs), and megadose.
- from the point of view of a healthy individual, discuss the advantages and disadvantages of using nutritional supplements.
- define the term calorie as it is commonly used, and state the amount of calories per gram of carbohydrate, protein, fat, and alcohol.
- describe the concepts of nutrient density and empty calories.

KEY NUTRIENTS

Nutrients are substances that supply the body with essential elements. These nutrients are necessary for:

- growth, maintenance, and repair of tissues;
- energy requirements;
- regulating body processes; and
- maintaining a constant internal environment.

More than 40 different nutrients are known to be needed for good health. Although all nutrients are important, some play a more important role than others. Those that play the most important role are known as the **key nutrients.** These nutrients, which are explained in greater detail in later chapters, include carbohydrates, proteins, fats, water, vitamins, and minerals.

Carbohydrates

Carbohydrates are the energy nutrients. They come primarily from plant sources.

Proteins

Proteins furnish energy and are the only nutrient capable of building body tissues. They come from both animal and plant sources.

Fats

Fats provide energy and fill other nutrient needs. They come from both animal and plant sources.

Water

Water is a key nutrient. It is an important part of most body structures and plays a major role in many bodily functions.

Vitamins

Vitamins are organic substances that are necessary in very small amounts for proper growth, development, and optimal health. **Organic** *substances* are composed of matter of plant or animal origin. Although vitamins are essential for good health, they are not an energy source.

Minerals

Minerals are inorganic substances that are necessary in very small amounts for proper growth, development, and optimal health. **Inorganic** *substances* are composed of matter other than plant or animal origin. Although minerals are essential for good health, they are not an energy source.

NUTRIENTS WORK INDIVIDUALLY AND TOGETHER

Good nutrition depends on an adequate supply of all of the essential nutrients.

- Each nutrient has a specific role in the building, maintaining, and functioning of the body.
- The role of one nutrient cannot be performed by other nutrients.

- The nutrients work together in an intricate, metabolic balance.
- A deficiency of one nutrient may interfere with the body's ability to utilize other nutrients.
- An extra supply of one nutrient cannot make up for a shortage of another nutrient.
- Best nutritional results do not come from concentrating on a single nutrient to the exclusion of other nutrients.
- All of the essential nutrients needed for good health are available through a well-balanced diet.

NUTRIENT NEEDS

Recommended Dietary Allowances (RDAs)

Recommended Dietary Allowances (RDAs) are established by the Food and Nutrition Board Commission on Life Sciences of the National Research Council. Their most recent recommendations were published in the book, *Recommended Dietary Allowances,* 10th Edition, which was published by the National Academy Press in 1989.

RDAs are recommendations for the specific average daily amount of each nutrient based on population groups classified by age and sex (Fig. 3-1). There are also categories for pregnant women and nursing mothers (lactating women). Throughout the text, the RDAs quoted for adults represent the 25- to 50-year-old age group.

RDAs are designed to meet the general basic needs of healthy individuals within each of these groups. They are not intended to cover individuals with special dietary needs, such as those which may be caused by illness, injury, or metabolic disorders.

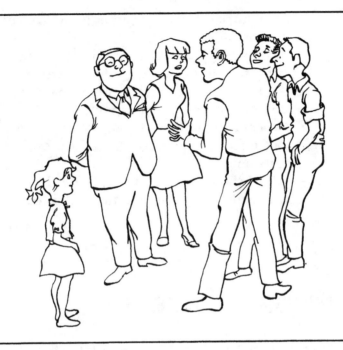

FIGURE 3-1 RDAs are nutritional recommendations for population groups based on age and sex.

Estimated Safe and Adequate Daily Dietary Intakes (ESIs)

When insufficient information is available to establish RDAs, **estimated safe and adequate daily dietary intakes (ESIs)** are used instead. This category includes the caution that upper levels in this range should not be habitually exceeded because of potential toxic effects. **Toxic** means poisonous

United States Recommended Daily Allowances (U.S. RDAs)

United States Recommended Daily Allowances (U.S. RDAs) are established by the United States Department of Agriculture (USDA). RDA values are established according to sex and age group needs. In contrast, the U.S. RDAs do not include this variation. Instead, they generally represent the highest value for any age group.

In the past, U.S. RDAs were used for purposes of comparison in nutritional labeling of food packages. The new labeling law is discussed in Chapter 8.

Reference Daily Intake (RDI)

Reference Daily Intake (RDI) is a new value that has been created to replace the current U.S. RDAs.

Megadoses

A **megadose** is defined as ten times the RDA for water-soluble vitamins and five times the RDA for fat-soluble vitamins. Vitamins and minerals taken in large quantities may be toxic or cause other health threats. Larger than recommended amounts of any of the nutrients should be taken only under qualified supervision.

NUTRIENTS AND SUPPLEMENTS

The best source of all essential nutrients is a well-balanced diet (Fig. 3-2). The guidelines outlined in Chapter 8 will help in the selection of the appropriate foods to achieve this goal.

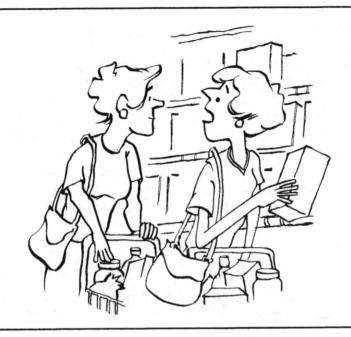

FIGURE 3-2 "Remember how much easier it was to shop when we thought nutrients came from vitamin pills?"

Although most people in the United States can get all of the nutrients they need from their daily dietary intake, many routinely take vitamin and mineral supplements. At best this may be a waste of money. At worst this action could actually be creating health risks.

The following general guidelines are helpful regarding the use of supplements:

- Vitamin and mineral supplements cannot replace food or turn a junk-food diet into a healthy one.
- Under current law, supplements are regarded as food not drugs. As such, they are not regulated by the Food and Drug Administration (FDA). This means that po-

tentially risky products are on the shelves without warning labels.

- For healthy individuals, vitamin and mineral supplements at or below the Recommended Dietary Allowances (RDAs) are considered to be safe but unnecessary.
- Taking excessive vitamins and minerals without medical supervision is risky and may be dangerous to your health.
- Taking large amounts of some isolated nutrients (such as specific B-complex vitamins) can upset the balance of other nutrients in the body. Unless prescribed by a physician for a specific reason avoid concentrated levels of specific vitamins.

Supplements may be necessary in the following situations:

- If you omit a major food group from your regular diet, you may need a supplement. However, a well-balanced diet with intake from each of the food groups is a better solution.
- If your usual diet contains less than 1,200 calories, you may need a multivitamin/mineral supplement.
- If you smoke, you may need to increase your intake of vitamin C. Smoking also increases the risk of many other disorders.
- Heavy alcohol consumption may increase your need for B-complex vitamins. It also provides many empty calories.
- Pregnant women and nursing mothers have special nutritional needs. They should consult their physicians about the need for a supplement.
- Women may need calcium supplements to help maintain strong bones. This need is discussed in Chapter 9.
- For many reasons, the elderly may need supplements. Their special needs are discussed in Chapter 9.

ENERGY NEEDS

The body converts food into the energy required to maintain the normal processes of life and to meet the demands of activity and growth. The body needs energy for three factors. These are: (1) energy for basal metabolism, (2) energy for physical activity, and (3) energy needed to digest and absorb the nutrients in food.

Basal metabolism is the least amount of energy needed to maintain essential life processes such as breathing, beating of the heart, circulation, and maintaining body temperature. Individual energy needs vary widely depending on age, sex, body weight, level of physical activity, and other specialized demands made upon the body.

Food intake can affect body weight in three ways:

1. Foods eaten must meet the body's energy and nutrient needs. To maintain a proper weight, food intake over time must reflect the body's energy needs.
2. If food intake exceeds the body's energy needs, the excess is stored as fat, and the individual gains weight.
3. If food intake does not meet the body's energy needs, changes in body weight or body composition will occur and may adversely affect health.

Calories

The calorie is the basic unit used to measure energy needs and energy use. One **calorie** (spelled with a small letter c) is the amount of heat required to raise the temperature of one gram of water by one degree Celsius. A **Calorie** (spelled with a capital C) is 1,000 times larger than the calorie. It is also known as a **kilocalorie** (kcal). The amount of energy in food is described in kilocalories. However, the term calorie (with a small c) is commonly used for this purpose.

The number of calories required per day to maintain ideal body weight depends upon factors such as sex, age, and activity level. The following will give you a general idea how much energy is required per day:

- An adult male (ages 23 to 50 years) weighing 154 pounds needs about 2,400 calories (kcals) per day.
- An adult female (ages 23 to 50 years) weighing 120 pounds needs about 2,000 calories (kcals) per day.

Calories Per Nutrient

As shown in Table 3-1, calories come in predictable quantities from the energy nutrients carbohydrates, proteins, and fat. (Alcohol, which is *not* a nutrient and does not contribute any nutrients to the diet, is included here because when consumed it is a major source of calories.)

Notice that the nutrient amounts are measured in terms of a single gram. The following examples will help you understand how this relates when foods are measured in a more familiar term such as a teaspoon:

- Four grams of sugar equals one teaspoon of sugar. This teaspoon of sugar contains 16 calories because each gram of carbohydrate contains four calories.
- Four grams of fat also equals one teaspoon. However, this teaspoon of fat contains 36 calories because each gram of fat contains nine calories.

Nutrient Density

When evaluating the amount of calories in a food item, it is also important to take into consideration what the food contributes to the body's nutritional needs. The term **nutrient density** describes how much nutritional value is re-

ceived per calorie. It is based on the concentration of each
nutrient per calorie of dietary energy.

For individuals whose energy needs are relatively low, or
for anyone on a restricted caloric intake, it is especially critical that foods of high nutrient density be selected to provide
an adequate supply of all nutrients. Skim milk is an excellent example of a food with high nutrient density. Although
one cup contains only 90 calories, it has 12 grams of carbohydrates, nine grams of protein, and only one gram of fat.
In addition, it is a good source of calcium and vitamins A
and D.

Empty Calories

Empty calories are contained in those foods that provide only energy and no other nutrients. Foods containing
only empty calories rate very low in terms of nutrient density. Empty calories are found in soft drinks, alcohol, and in
foods with high sugar and fat contents.

1 gram of **carbohydrate**	4 calories
1 gram of **protein**	4 calories
1 gram of **fat**	9 calories
1 gram of **alcohol**	7 calories

TABLE 3-1 Calories per gram of Energy Nutrient

REVIEW EXERCISES _____

MULTIPLE CHOICE

Circle the correct answer for each question.

1. _____ are the energy nutrients that come primarily from plant sources.

   a) Carbohydrates
   b) Minerals
   c) Vitamins

2. Extra quantities of one nutrient _____ make up for a deficiency of another nutrient.

   a) can
   b) cannot

3. A megadose is defined as _____ times the RDA for water-soluble vitamins.

   a)   5
   b) 10
   c) 100

4. Minerals are _____ substances that are composed of matter other than of plant or animal origin.

   a) inorganic
   b) organic
   c) synthetic

5. _____ are organic substances which are necessary in very small amounts for proper growth, development, and optimal health.

   a) Minerals
   b) Proteins
   c) Vitamins

6. An adequate supply of vitamin and mineral supplements _____ make up for deficiencies in a junk-food diet.

   a) can
   b) cannot

7. _____ are the only nutrients capable of building body tissue.

   a) Carbohydrates
   b) Fats
   c) Proteins

8. When insufficient information is available to establish RDAs, _____ are used instead.

   a) estimated safe and adequate daily dietary intakes (ESIs)
   b) reference daily intakes (RDIs)
   c) United States recommended daily allowances (U.S. RDAs)

9. Under current law, vitamin and mineral supplements are regarded as _____.

   a) drugs
   b) food
   c) therapeutics

10. Four grams of fat contains _____ calories.

    a) 16
    b) 28
    c) 36

SUGGESTED CLASS ACTIVITY

Begin collecting the "Nutrition Information" portion from food labels. You will need these for use with later chapters.

Read the label information on at least one type of vitamin and mineral supplement. What portions of the RDAs does this supplement supply? Be prepared to discuss whether or not taking this supplement is a good idea for a healthy young adult.

Discuss in class whether there should be additional controls placed on the types of claims that may be made by food supplements.

CHAPTER 4

CARBOHYDRATES

OBJECTIVES

After studying this chapter, you should be able to:

- describe the major functions of carbohydrates.
- differentiate between complex and refined carbohydrates and name sources of each.
- name the three classifications of carbohydrates based on the number of molecules of sugar, and name at least one form of sugar in each group.
- differentiate between glucose and glycogen and describe how excess glucose is stored.
- describe the following sweeteners: sucrose, confectioner's sugar, brown sugar, dextrose, corn sweetener, fructose, honey, invert sugar, maple syrup, molasses, raw sugar, and turbinado.
- describe how sugar alcohols differ from other sugars.
- name three nonnutritive sweeteners.
- describe the major functions of fiber and list at least three good sources of fiber.

MAJOR FUNCTIONS OF CARBOHYDRATES

The primary function of **carbohydrates** is to provide the energy necessary to support life. Under normal circumstances, carbohydrates supply the fuel to meet about two-thirds of an individual's total energy needs. The remaining energy needs are filled by other food sources.

Additional functions of carbohydrates are listed below.

- Carbohydrates furnish the dietary fiber needed for normal **peristalsis** (a series of wave-like contractions that move food through the intestines) and the elimination of solid body waste. (Fiber is discussed later in this chapter.)
- Carbohydrates affect food consumption by providing sweetness and making food taste better.
- Carbohydrates supply other vital nutrients, such as vitamins and minerals.
- Carbohydrates are needed to "burn" fats completely. Acidosis results when there are not enough carbohydrates present to completely burn these fats. **Acidosis** is characterized by an abnormally high level of acid in the blood, or by a decrease in the alkali reserve in the body.

If there are not enough carbohydrates present in the diet, the body must use protein as an energy source. This prevents protein from performing its primary functions of building and repairing body tissues.

A diet totally lacking in carbohydrates is likely to lead to ketosis, excessive breakdown of tissue protein, loss of sodium, and involuntary dehydration. **Ketosis** is a clinical condition that is characterized by a sweetish acetone odor of the breath.

SOURCES OF CARBOHYDRATES

Carbohydrates come primarily from plant sources and are described as being either complex or refined (Fig. 4-1).

Complex Carbohydrates

In nature, **complex carbohydrates** are mainly vegetable products such as grains, vegetables, and fruits. Milk and dairy products contain carbohydrates in the form of lactose (milk sugar).

In addition to containing naturally occurring sugars, complex carbohydrates also provide other nutrients, particularly vitamins and minerals.

Refined Carbohydrates

Refined carbohydrates include foods such as sugar, syrup, jelly, bread, cookies, cakes, soft drinks, and other sweets. Alcohol is a refined substance that the body processes as a carbohydrate.

In contrast to complex carbohydrates, most refined carbohydrates do not provide additional nutrients. Instead most refined nutrients supply only empty calories.

CLASSIFICATION OF CARBOHYDRATES

All carbohydrates are made up of one or more molecules of sugar. Based on this structure, carbohydrates are classified as monosaccharides (single sugars), disaccharides (double sugars), and polysaccharides (multiple sugars as found in complex carbohydrates).

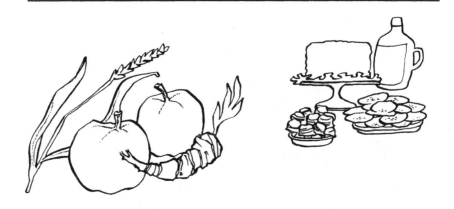

COMPLEX CARBOHYDRATES   REFINED CARBOHYDRATES

FIGURE 4-1   Carbohydrates may be either complex or
refined.

Monosaccharides

The **monosaccharides** (single sugars) are the simplest
form of carbohydrate. They are the form most readily utilized by the body. The monosaccharides include **glucose,
fructose,** and **galactose.**

Glucose

Glucose, which is also known as **dextrose,** is the form
of sugar found in some foods. It is also the form of sugar that
is found in the blood. This form is discussed later in this
chapter.

Fructose

Fructose, which is also known as **fruit sugar** or
levulose, is the sweetest of all sugars. It is found in ripe

fruit, juices, and honey. The liver readily converts fructose into glucose.

Galactose

Galactose is less soluble and not as sweet as glucose; however, the liver readily converts galactose into glucose.

Disaccharides

The **disaccharides** (double sugars) must be broken down into the simpler monosaccharide form before they can be utilized by the body. The disaccharides include **sucrose, lactose,** and **maltose.**

Sucrose

Sucrose, which is commonly known as **table sugar,** is a combination of glucose and fructose.

Lactose

Lactose, which is also known as **milk sugar,** is found in milk and is the only sugar that is not from plant sources. Lactose is less soluble than sucrose and is not as sweet. However, it remains in the intestines longer than other sugars and encourages the growth of certain useful bacteria.

Maltose

Maltose is formed from the amylase enzyme breakdown of starch in the small intestine.

Polysaccharides

The **polysaccharides** are the more complex carbohydrates. They include **starch, glycogen,** and **cellulose.**

Starch

Starch, which comes from plants, is nutritionally the most important carbohydrate. During digestion the body breaks starch into simpler forms. Because this takes longer than the digestion of monosaccharides and disaccharides the energy from these foods is released more slowly into the body.

Glycogen

Glycogen is the equivalent of starch but from animal sources.

Cellulose

Cellulose is a polysaccharide vegetable fiber that is not digested by humans.

GLUCOSE AND GLYCOGEN

Glucose

Glucose is the form of sugar normally found in the blood. In this form it is also known as **blood sugar.** Glucose is produced by the body through the digestive processing of carbohydrates. It is absorbed into the bloodstream from the small intestine and is utilized directly by the tissues as a source of energy.

Glycogen

If the energy is not needed by the body, it is stored in the liver and muscles as **glycogen.** When the body needs energy, this stored glycogen is broken down to glucose and released into the bloodstream.

When a meal provides more glucose than the tissues can use for energy, and the glycogen reserve needs of the liver and muscles have been satisfied, the excess glucose is turned into fat and deposited as adipose (fat) tissues throughout the body.

MORE ABOUT SUGARS

The U.S. Department of Agriculture estimates that Americans consume about 127 pounds of caloric sweeteners (sucrose and corn sweeteners) per year. Most sweeteners consumed are in manufactured foods and beverages. Table 4-1 shows the sugar content of popular foods.

Because so many types of sweeteners are available and are used in such a wide variety of products, most of us are not aware of how much we actually consume each day. These sugars are virtually all empty calories because few, if any, additional nutrients are provided.

The following are some of the types of sugar and sweeteners that may be added to foods:

- **Sucrose** (white, refined table sugar) is produced commercially by refining juice from the sugar cane or sugar beet plant.
- **Confectioner's sugar** (powdered sugar) is a powdery form of sugar.
- **Brown sugar** consists of sucrose crystals colored with molasses syrup. It is 91 to 96 percent sucrose.
- **Dextrose,** which is also known as **glucose** or **corn sugar,** is sugar made from cornstarch.
- **Corn sweetener** is a liquid sugar made from the breakdown of cornstarch. On a food label the term "corn sweeteners" may include various syrups, such as dextrose, that are derived from corn.

Food Source	Serving Size	Sugar Content*
Soft drinks (regular)	12 ounces	37.85 grams
Milk chocolate	1 ounce	15.3 grams
Hard candy	1 ounce	18.7 grams
Apple, medium raw	1 medium	18.4 grams
Banana, medium	1 medium	17.8 grams
Froot Loops cereal	1 ounce	13.9 grams
Shredded Wheat cereal	1 ounce	0.1 grams
Granola bar	1.8 ounce	19.7 grams
Fastfood "shake"	1 serving	52.2 grams
Raisins, dried	2/3 cup	65.0 grams
Spaghetti sauce	4 ounces	12.4 grams
Tomato soup (canned)	1 serving	12.6 grams
Broccoli, raw	1/2 cup	0.7 grams

* *Reminder*: four grams of sugar equals one teaspoon of sugar.

TABLE 4-1 Sugar Content of Popular Foods

- **Corn syrup** is a syrup made by the partial breakdown of cornstarch. High fructose corn syrups may be referred to by the abbreviation HFCS.
- **Fructose,** also known as **levulose,** is sweeter than sucrose. Fructose is used as a substitute for sucrose in some products that advertise themselves as being "lower in calories." Unlike other sugars, fructose doesn't require insulin to get into the liver and body cells. This is an advantage for diabetics who cannot produce insulin in adequate amounts.
- **Fruit juice concentrate,** particularly apple juice concentrate, is used as the sweetener in many foods

such as canned fruits that list themselves as having "no sugar added."

- **Honey** contains slightly more fructose than glucose and smaller amounts of other sugars (plus water). It also has some minerals that are present in such tiny amounts that they have little significance in human nutrition. Because it is produced by bees from various sources honey may also contain substances which may trigger allergic reactions in some individuals.

- **Invert sugar,** also known as **total invert sugar,** is a mixture of glucose and fructose. It is sold only in liquid form and is sweeter than sucrose. It helps prolong the freshness of baked goods and confections and is useful in preventing food shrinkage.

- **Maple syrup** is a syrup made from the sap of the sugar maple tree. Many of these syrups also contain corn syrup or other sweeteners; however, these additives must be listed on the label.

- **Molasses** is the syrup that is separated from raw sugar during processing. It contains a variety of sugars and small amounts of calcium, iron, potassium, and B-complex vitamins plus water. The darker molasses is nutritionally superior, and blackstrap molasses is best. However, molasses should still be thought of primarily as a form of sugar.

- **Raw sugar** is an intermediate product in the refining process. It is composed of sugar crystals covered with a syrup that may contain undesirable materials such as dirt, insect fragments, and plant debris. Because of these impurities, the use of raw sugar is prohibited in the United States.

- **Turbinado,** which is generally off-white in color, is partially refined sugar; however, it is often marketed as "raw sugar."

Sugar Alcohols

Sugar alcohols are synthetic sweetening products made from sugars or cellulose. The digestive system metabolizes these more slowly than it does sugar; however, they are eventually used by the body as sugar.

The most popular sugar alcohols are **sorbitol, mannitol,** and **xylitol.** These are sometimes used in products such as sugarless chewing gum because they are not converted into sugar in the mouth.

Nonnutritive Sweeteners

Nonnutritive sweeteners are sweetening agents that do not contribute nutrients or significant calories to the diet. The use of nonnutritive sweeteners is one way to limit the intake of empty calories in the diet.

The following are nonnutritive sweeteners:

- **Saccharin** is a nonnutritive sweetener that is 500 times sweeter than sucrose.
- **Aspartame** is a nonnutritive sweetener that is 180 times sweeter than sucrose.
- **Cyclamates** are nonnutritive sweeteners that are 50 times sweeter than sucrose; however, their use is banned in the United States.

DIETARY FIBER

Dietary fiber is defined as those components of carbohydrates that are indigestible. In human food these include **cellulose, hemicellulose, lignin, pectin, pentosan,** and **gum.**

Major Functions of Fiber

Fiber is useful to the body for the following reasons:

- Fiber helps provide the bulk necessary to assure normal peristalsis and the elimination of solid body waste.
- The pectins and gums in dietary fiber are important factors in how the body handles fats, cholesterol, and carbohydrates.
- Fiber yields few, if any, calories. Many fibrous foods, especially fruits and vegetables, are low in calories.
- Adequate fiber in the diet has been shown to reduce the risk of some diseases.

Sources of Fiber

In general, high-fiber foods are complex carbohydrates such as whole-grain versions of bread, cereal, and pasta; brown rice; fruits and vegetables; and dried beans, nuts, and seeds. Figure 4-2 and Table 4-2 show the dietary fiber content of popular foods. Notice that meat is not a good source of fiber.

Cooking, canning, and freezing do not seem to have any significant impact on food's natural fiber content. However, when fruits or vegetables are made into juices most of their fiber is generally discarded.

Refined carbohydrates are *not* a good source of fiber (Fig. 4-2). Foods low in fiber also include dairy products, meats, fish, poultry, refined grain products, sweeteners, fats, and oils.

Soluble Fiber

Soluble fiber is a type of dietary fiber which, when combined with a diet low in saturated fat, may be useful in

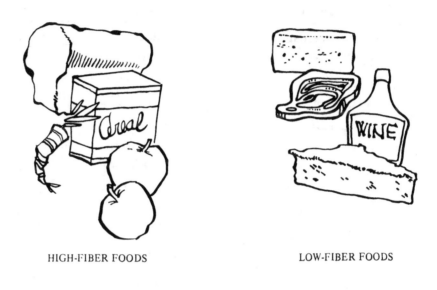

HIGH-FIBER FOODS   LOW-FIBER FOODS

FIGURE 4-2 Foods vary in their fiber content.

reducing blood cholesterol. Soluble fiber is found in grains such as psyllium, oats, and barley; in fruits such as prunes and apples; and in beans such as kidney beans.

Insoluble Fiber

Insoluble fiber, which is found primarily in wheat bran and whole grains, is good for the digestive system and may help protect against colon cancer.

Fiber Requirements

Fiber is a very important part of a well-balanced diet; however, it is not considered to be an essential nutrient

Food Source	Serving Size (calories)	Dietary Fiber
All-Bran cereal	1 ounce (71)	8.5 grams
Apple, raw	1 medium (80)	4.2 grams
Beef, baked ground lean	3-1/2 ounces (270)	0.0 grams
Broccoli, raw	1/2 cup (12)	0.6 grams
Carrot, raw	1 medium (30)	1.6 grams
Corn, cooked	1/2 cup (90)	2.1 grams
Navy beans, cooked	1/2 cup (130)	6.5 grams
Peanuts	1 ounce (160)	2.1 grams
Prunes, dried	1 cup (390)	10.9 grams
Raspberries, fresh	1 cup (60)	5.8 grams
Spinach, raw	1/2 cup (6)	1.1 grams

TABLE 4-2   Dietary Fiber Content of Popular Foods

because people can survive without fiber in their diet. Nutritionists generally recommend a dietary intake of fiber from both sources of 25 to 35 grams per day.

Low Fiber Intake

Studies suggest that cancer of the colon may be related to a low fiber intake. Low fiber intake has also been implicated in cardiovascular disease.

Excessive Fiber Intake

Taking fiber supplements, or suddenly switching to a high-fiber diet can be risky because high dietary fiber intake may reduce the absorption of minerals such as calcium, iron, and zinc. Also, a sudden increase in dietary fiber may cause flatulence (gas), cramps, constipation, and diarrhea.

For these reasons it is desirable to gradually increase fiber from a wide variety of natural sources and to drink plenty of fluids.

REVIEW EXERCISES _____

MULTIPLE CHOICE

Circle the correct answer for each question.

1. _____ is commonly known as table sugar.

   a) Dextrose
   b) Glucose
   c) Sucrose

2. Glucose is also known as _____.

   a) blood sugar
   b) levulose
   c) raffinose

3. The simplest form of carbohydrate is called _____.

   a) disaccharide
   b) monosaccharide
   c) polysaccharide

4. When the body needs energy, the stored _____ is broken down to glucose and released into the bloodstream.

   a) cellulose
   b) glycogen
   c) sucrose

5. The generally recommended dietary fiber intake is _____ grams per day.

   a) 15 to 25
   b) 25 to 35
   c) 35 to 50

6. _____ fiber may be helpful in reducing blood cholesterol.

   a) Insoluble
   b) Soluble

7. Fructose is a _____ form of carbohydrate.

   a) disaccharide
   b) monosaccharide
   c) polysaccharide

8. The primary function of carbohydrates is to _____.

   a) build body tissues
   b) repair body tissues
   c) supply fuel for energy needs

9. Raw vegetables contain _____ carbohydrates.

   a) complex
   b) refined

10. _____ results when there are not enough carbohydrates present to completely burn the fats in the diet.

    a) Acidosis
    b) Involuntary dehydration
    c) Ketosis

SUGGESTED CLASS ACTIVITY

Review Table 4-1 and discuss which foods are empty calories, which are likely to be high in fat, and which provide important additional nutrients.

Review Table 4-2 and discuss which foods would be the best fiber source for the least amount of calories.

Make a list of the foods you ate yesterday and have eaten so far today. Identify the carbohydrates you ate during this period. Separate these into complex carbohydrates (grains, fruits, vegetables) and refined carbohydrates (cake, cookies, baked goods, candy, soda, etc.).

This is far from a complete dietary analysis; however, review your figures and try to estimate if you are getting too many of your calories from refined carbohydrates. Also, try to estimate if you are consuming enough dietary fiber to meet the recommended daily amounts.

CHAPTER 5

PROTEINS, FATS, AND WATER

OBJECTIVES

After studying this chapter, you should be able to:

- state the major functions of proteins and list major sources of protein.
- differentiate between essential and nonessential amino acids.
- differentiate between complete and incomplete proteins, and describe the role of complementary proteins.
- state the major functions of fats.
- discuss the differences between saturated and unsaturated fats and identify dietary sources of each.
- describe the role of essential fatty acids and identify their primary sources.
- describe the major functions and sources of water.

PROTEINS

Major Functions of Proteins

Proteins form the fundamental structural materials of every body cell. The primary functions of proteins are to repair worn-out or wasted tissue and to build new tissue. Proteins are important because they are the only nutrients that can carry out these functions.

Proteins are a normal part of all body fluids except bile and urine. As such, proteins are active in regulating osmotic pressures within body fluids to maintain normal circulation and water balance.

Proteins are also used by the body in manufacturing hormones and enzymes and in building antibodies to fight infections. In addition, proteins transport oxygen and nutrients in the blood and are essential to the clotting of blood.

Proteins are broken down into component parts in the digestive tract and are then absorbed into the bloodstream. In the tissues new proteins are built from these components. Dietary protein, however, cannot be stored by the body; it requires a new supply daily.

Daily Requirements of Proteins

If the diet does not supply adequate calories from other sources, dietary protein may be burned to furnish heat and energy to the body. However, the body's energy needs are best met from carbohydrate sources.

When protein is severely deficient relative to calories, kwashiorkor may develop. **Kwashiorkor,** also known as **protein-calorie malnutrition,** is a nutritional deficiency disease caused by an inadequate intake of protein. Kwashiorkor is rarely seen in the United States where most people eat excessive amounts of protein; however, it is a major problem in developing countries where food shortages are severe.

Too much protein in the diet puts a strain on the liver and kidneys which must process the excess. Excessive protein intake also increases the urinary excretion of calcium. This in turn reduces the amount of calcium available for use by the body.

The RDA for protein for adult males is 63 grams per day. For adult females it is 50 grams per day.

Sources of Proteins

Protein sources include meat, fish, poultry, eggs, milk and dairy products, dried beans and peas, peanut butter, nuts, bread and cereal (Fig. 5-1). Table 5-1 shows the protein and fat content of popular foods.

Amino Acids

Proteins differ in nutritive value because they differ in their amino acid composition. **Amino acids** are the building blocks of protein. They are defined as the fundamental structural units of proteins. They are nitrogen-containing chemicals that are strung together in ever-larger units until a complete protein is formed. The order of these amino acid molecules and the particular combination of amino acids determine the property of the resulting protein.

Ordinarily all 22 of the known amino acids are required for the synthesis (manufacture) of tissue proteins. The absence of any one amino acid could prevent this synthesis.

The body can synthesize the majority of these amino acids or obtain them from the diet; however, some amino acids cannot be synthesized in amounts adequate for metabolic needs.

Those amino acids that can be synthesized by the body in adequate quantities are called **nonessential amino acids.** Those amino acids that are needed, but not synthe-

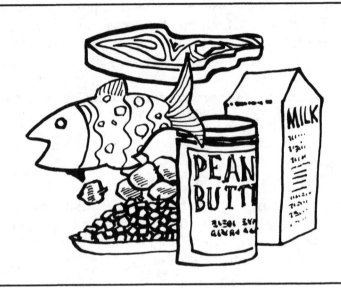

FIGURE 5-1 Examples of protein sources.

sized by the body, are termed **essential amino acids.** If
health is to be maintained, these essential amino acids must
be supplied by the diet.

Experts place the following amino acids in the essential
amino acid category:

- tryptophan,
- threonine,
- isoleucine,
- leucine,
- lysine,
- methionine,
- phenylalanine,
- valine,
- histidine, and
- arginine.

Food	Serving (calories)	Protein (gram)	Fat (gram)
Chicken, dark meat (roasted without skin)	3 ounces (174)	17	8
Chicken, light meat (roasted without skin)	3 ounces (144)	26	7
Milk, skim	1 cup (90)	8	<1
Milk, whole	1 cup (160)	8	9
Pasta, cooked (no sauce)	1/2 cup (100)	3	<1
Peanut butter	2 tbs (190)	8	16
Shrimp, steamed	4 large (20)	5	<1
Sirloin steak, lean (broiled)	3 ounces (240)	23	15

TABLE 5-1 Protein and Fat Content of Popular Foods

Complete and Incomplete Proteins

A **complete protein** is a food protein that contains all of the essential amino acids in significant amounts and in proportions fairly similar to those found in body protein. Complete proteins can supply the needs of the body for maintenance, repair, and growth. Complete proteins are derived from animal foods such as meat, fish, eggs, milk, and cheese. Gelatin is the only food taken from an animal source that is *not* a complete protein.

An **incomplete protein** is a protein lacking one or more of the essential amino acids or supplying too little of an essential amino acid to support health. These are food proteins that, by themselves, cannot perform the functions of synthesis. The incomplete proteins are derived from plant foods such as grains, peas, nuts, beans, and vegetables.

Complementary Proteins

Complementary proteins are incomplete proteins from different sources that work together to supply missing or incomplete amino acids. For example, corn complements beans. This pairing of complementary incomplete proteins enables the proteins to function as effectively as complete proteins. It is through this skillful combination of incomplete proteins that vegetarians are able to obtain an adequate supply of protein in their diets.

FATS

Major Functions of Fats

Fats are normal structural components of every cell wall and every membrane within a cell. They carry and facilitate absorption of the fat-soluble vitamins A, D, E, and K. Fats also provide essential fatty acids.

Body fats help to maintain body temperature by insulating against cold. They also act as a cushion mechanism for protecting vital organs such as the kidneys and reproductive organs. Without a minimal level of body fat, a woman's sex-hormone balance and menstrual cycle are disrupted. **Amenorrhea,** which is an absence of menstruation, may result.

Fats provide a large amount of energy in a small amount

of food. They also give a sensation of fullness because they stay in the stomach longer than protein or carbohydrates and digest relatively slowly in the intestines.

Although fats do serve an important function, no daily servings are recommended. This is because our daily fat requirements are filled by fats contained in the other foods we eat.

Fats of all kinds have been implicated in heart disease and other health problems. In fact, excess dietary fats are considered to be one of the major health problems in the United States today.

Sources of Fats

Fats come from animal and vegetable sources such as meats; milk, cream, butter, and cheese; cooking and salad oils and dressings; and nuts and nut products such as peanut butter.

Table 5-1 shows the protein and fat content of popular foods. Figure 5-2 illustrates one way to reduce fat consumption without compromising nutrient value.

Dietary Fats

About 95 percent of dietary fat consists of complex molecules called **triglycerides** which in turn make up smaller substances called **fatty acids.** All animal and vegetable fats are composed of glycerol (an alcohol) attached to fatty-acid chains made up of carbon, hydrogen, and oxygen atoms.

Fatty acids come in two types: saturated and unsaturated. Simply put, **saturated fats** have a full complement of hydrogen atoms; **unsaturated fats** are short some hydrogen atoms along their fatty-acid chains.

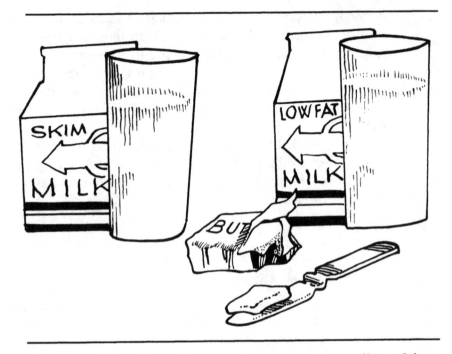

FIGURE 5-2   The difference between skim milk and low fat milk is one pat of butter. The difference between skim milk and whole milk is two pats of butter.

Saturated Fats

Saturated fats come primarily from animal food products such as butter, whole milk, bacon, luncheon meats, and fatty meats. Saturated fats are naturally hard at room temperature.

Palm oil and coconut oil are examples of saturated fats from plant sources. Saturated fats are also found in microwave popcorn, nondairy creamers, and granola-type cereal.

Saturated fats increase the amount of cholesterol in the blood and are *not* an essential part of the diet.

Unsaturated Fats

Unsaturated fats are further divided into two categories: **monounsaturated** and **polyunsaturated,** depending on the number of hydrogen atoms missing along the chain.

Monounsaturated fats, such as olive oil, peanut oil, and canola oil are primarily oleic acid. These fats are thought to have a neutral or slightly beneficial effect on blood cholesterol.

Polyunsaturated fats are found in most vegetable oils such as corn, cottonseed, sunflower, safflower, and soybean. These fats are sometimes listed as **PUFA** which stands for polyunsaturated fatty acids.

Oils high in polyunsaturated fats tend to lower the serum cholesterol level. Serum cholesterol is discussed further in Chapter 9.

Table 5-2 shows the relative amounts of different types of fats in commonly used plant oils. Butter is included in the table to show the relative amounts of fats in an animal product.

Oil	Saturated	Polyunsaturated	Monounsaturated
Olive	14%	9%	77%
Canola	6%	36%	58%
Peanut	18%	38%	48%
Corn	13%	62%	25%
Soybean	15%	61%	24%
Safflower	9%	78%	13%
Butter	66%	4%	30% butterfat

TABLE 5-2 What's in an Oil?

Hydrogenated Oils

Hydrogenation is the process whereby oils are changed into solid fats at room temperature. (Oils are fats that are naturally liquid at room temperature.) To "solidify" oils (such as soybean oil, corn, or sunflower), hydrogen atoms are forced into the unsaturated fatty-acid chains. This makes unsaturated fatty acids more saturated but stops short of complete saturation. The resulting chain, which is still unsaturated, is called a **trans-fatty acid.**

These changes cause hydrogenated oils to be higher in saturated fat content than the oils they are made from. For example, the saturation of all-vegetable shortening ranges from 25 to 30 percent saturated fat.

Essential Fatty Acids

Essential Fatty Acids (EFAs) are polyunsaturated fatty acids required by the body.

Linoleic and **arachidonic acids** are essential fatty acids needed by the body for normal growth and healthy skin. They also have a role in reducing the amount of cholesterol in the blood. Linoleic acid is necessary for the body to utilize fats properly. Both fatty acids are found primarily in the polyunsaturated fats of vegetable oils including corn, cottonseed, peanut, soybean, and safflower.

WATER

Major Functions of Water

Water is sometimes referred to as the forgotten nutrient, yet it is second only to oxygen as being essential for life. Humans can live longer without food than without water.

Chemical reactions between substances take place only when they are in a solution. Water promotes body processes by acting as a solvent and thereby making chemical reactions possible.

Water also helps to build tissue. Bone is one-third water, muscle is two-thirds water, and whole blood is four-fifths water.

Water helps to regulate body temperature by transporting heat from one part to another. This aids in equalizing body temperature. Furthermore, water evaporated from the skin and lungs rids the body of excess heat.

The preservation of the body's fluid balance depends on thirst stimulus and renal (kidney) compensatory mechanisms. The distribution of water inside and outside the cells depends on adequate protein and balanced mineral intake. Sodium and potassium are the minerals primarily responsible for water balance.

Sources of Water

The sources of body water are the liquids we drink, the water in our food, and the water formed by oxidation of our food. However, coffee, tea, and alcohol are diuretics. A **diuretic** causes water to be excreted by the kidneys.

If the loss of water exceeds the intake, the patient may become dehydrated. **Dehydration** means the loss of water from the body. Continued or severe dehydration can be fatal.

REVIEW EXERCISES _____

MULTIPLE CHOICE

Circle the correct answer for each question.

1. _____ are the building blocks of protein.

   a) Amino acids
   b) Linoleic acids
   c) Polyunsaturated fats

2. _____ fats increase the amount of cholesterol in the blood.

   a) Monounsaturated
   b) Polyunsaturated
   c) Saturated

3. Based on the information in Table 5-1, a 3-ounce serving of steak provides almost _____ percent of a woman's RDA for protein.

   a) 1/4
   b) 1/2
   c) 100

4. This serving of steak has 15 grams of fat. Based on what you learned in Chapter 2 about calories per gram of specific nutrients, _____ calories in this steak come from fat.

   a) 60
   b) 105
   c) 135

5. _____ are used by the body in building antibodies to fight infections.

a) Amino acids
b) Saturated fats
c) Proteins

6. If a food is lacking an essential amino acid, the body _____ able to manufacture the missing component.

a) is
b) is not

7. Saturated fats are often naturally hard at room temperature and come primarily from _____ sources.

a) animal
b) manufactured
c) vegetable

8. Linoleic and arachidonic acids are _____ needed by the body for normal growth and healthy skin.

a) essential fatty acids
b) trans-fatty acids
c) triglycerides

9. Bone consists of _____ water.

a) 1/8
b) 1/4
c) 1/3

10. A _____ causes water to be excreted by the kidneys.

    a) diuretic
    b) hydrogenation
    c) tryptophan

SUGGESTED CLASS ACTIVITY

Start gathering information on the nutritional values in some fast foods such as a cheeseburger, fries, or chicken nuggets. (Many fast-food chains have this information readily available. Others will provide it if you ask.)

Review the table below and calculate the number of calories from fat in each dish. Be prepared to discuss the following in class.

- Which meal has the lowest total number of calories?
- Which meal has the highest total number of calories?
- Which meal has the lowest number of calories from fat?
- Which meal has the highest number of calories from fat?
- Is there always a direct relationship between the number of calories in a meal and the amount of fat that is in the meal?

Frozen Dinner	Calories	Fat (grams)	Calories from fat
Chicken enchiladas	310	9	
Chicken polynesian	190	5	
Ham & asparagus au gratin	300	9	
Southern baked chicken	170	7	

CHAPTER 6

VITAMINS

OBJECTIVES _____

After studying this chapter, you should be able to:

- describe the function of vitamins in human nutrition.
- compare a microgram with a milligram and an international unit with a retinol unit.
- define the terms antioxidant and precursor.
- differentiate between fat-and water-soluble vitamins and list the vitamins in each group.
- describe the major role and sources for each vitamin.

THE FUNCTIONS OF VITAMINS

Vitamins are organic substances that are necessary in minute amounts for proper growth, development, and optimal health. Table 6-1 lists the vitamins.

The major functions of vitamins as a group include:

- assisting the body in the processing of other nutrients (proteins, fats, carbohydrates, and minerals).
- participating in the formation of blood cells, hormones, genetic material, and nervous system chemicals.
- acting as coenzymes to assist enzymes in carrying out their functions. The function of enzymes is explained in Chapter 2.

Antioxidants

An **antioxidant** is a substance that slows the deterioration of materials through the oxidation process. In addition

Fat-Soluble Vitamins	Water-Soluble Vitamins
Vitamin A	Vitamin C
Vitamin D	Thiamin (vitamin B_1)
Vitamin E	Riboflavin (vitamin B_2)
Vitamin K	Niacin (vitamin B_2)
	Vitamin B_6
	Folic acid (folacin)
	Vitamin B_{12}
	Biotin
	Pantothenic acid

TABLE 6-1   Fat-soluble and water-soluble vitamins

to their other functions, vitamins C and E and **beta carotene** (the precursor of vitamin A) appear to play a protective role as antioxidants. A **precursor** is a substance from which another substance is formed. This means that the body is able to convert beta carotene into vitamin A as needed.

The role of these nutrients as antioxidants is not yet fully understood; however, apparently they are able to inactivate harmful molecules that can damage cells. These destructive molecules, which are known as *oxygen-free radicals,* are a normal by-product of metabolism in cells. Toxic molecules are also created in the body by exposure to sunlight, x-rays, ozone, tobacco smoke, car exhaust, and other environmental pollutants.

DAILY VITAMIN NEEDS

Vitamins are so important that we cannot live without them. Yet they are required in such small amounts that all the needed vitamins together add up to about an eighth of a teaspoon per day. Daily requirements for vitamins are expressed as **Recommended Dietary Allowances (RDAs)** or as **estimated safe and adequate daily dietary intakes (ESIs).** These terms are explained in Chapter 3.

Quantities of Vitamins

Quantities of vitamins may be expressed in **milligrams** (mg), **micrograms** (mcg), **retinol equivalents** (REs), or **international units** (IUs). One microgram is one-thousandth (1/1000) of a milligram. Five international units (IU) equal one retinol equivalent (RE).

FAT-SOLUBLE VITAMINS

The **fat-soluble vitamins** are A, D, E, and K. These vitamins are absorbed through the intestinal membranes with the aid of fats in the diet or bile produced by the liver. They are not destroyed by cooking.

Since fat-soluble vitamins are stored in body fat, it is not essential to consume them daily. However, because they are stored in the body, excessive amounts can build to toxic levels.

Vitamin A

Major Roles Of Vitamin A

Vitamin A, which is also known as **retinol,** helps build and maintain healthy tissues (skin, hair, nails, mucous membranes). Vitamin A also promotes good vision and helps maintain the immune system.

The RDA for vitamin A is expressed in retinol equivalent (RE) units. For an adult male the RDA is 1,000 RE; for an adult female the RDA is 800 RE.

Sources of Vitamin A

Vitamin A from food sources is known as **preformed vitamin A.** It is available from animal sources such as liver, fish liver oils, eggs, and fortified whole milk. In this situation, **fortified** means that vitamins A and D have been added to the milk.

Beta carotene, a precursor of vitamin A, is found in yellow and dark-green leafy vegetables and fruits such as broccoli, spinach, carrots, sweet potatoes, squash, apricots, and cantaloupe.

Some nutritionists recommend five to six milligrams of

beta carotene a day. This requirement is easily met by eating a single carrot or half a cantaloupe.

Signs of Vitamin A Deficiency

A deficiency of vitamin A can cause **night blindness,** dryness of the eyes, and serious changes in the cornea. It may also cause rough skin and mucous membranes, poor dental development, impairment of growth and reproduction, and decreased resistance to infection.

When deficiencies occur they are most likely to be found in children under five years of age due to insufficient dietary intake. They may also occur in adults as a result of chronic fat malabsorption.

Vitamin A Megadose Risks

Megadoses of vitamin A can result in toxic manifestations including double vision, headaches, vomiting, diarrhea, skin rashes, hair loss, liver damage, joint pain, abnormal bone growth, insomnia, extreme fatigue, menstrual irregularities, birth defects, and injury to the brain and nervous systems.

Vitamin D

Major Roles of Vitamin D

Vitamin D assists in the absorption and use of calcium and phosphorus. Therefore, it is essential for the formation and maintenance of strong bones and teeth. The RDA for vitamin D for adult males and females is five micrograms.

Sources of Vitamin D

The major food source of vitamin D is fortified milk products. Vitamin D is also produced by the body following exposure to sunlight.

Signs of Vitamin D Deficiency

Rickets is caused by a deficiency of vitamin D, especially in infancy and childhood. **Rickets** is a condition in which there is a disturbance in the normal ossification (hardening) of the bones. This may result in disturbances of growth with associated skeletal deformities and frequent fractures.

In adults, a lack of vitamin D may result in **hypocalcemia** (an abnormally low level of calcium in the blood), **osteomalacia** (abnormal softening of the bones), or **osteoporosis** (an abnormal loss of bone density resulting in weak, brittle bones).

Vitamin D Megadose Risks

In infants, vitamin D megadoses may cause calcium deposits in the kidneys and excessive calcium in the blood. In adults, vitamin D megadoses are potentially toxic and may result in irreversible kidney and cardiovascular damage.

Vitamin E

Major Roles of Vitamin E

Vitamin E aids in the formation of red blood cells, muscles, and other tissues. It is also an antioxidant. The RDA for vitamin E for an adult male is 10 milligrams; for an adult female it is eight milligrams.

Sources of Vitamin E

Vitamin E is found in vegetable oils (soybean, corn, cottonseed, and safflower) and in products such as margarine that are made from these oils.

Signs of Vitamin E Deficiency

Vitamin E deficiency is rare. It is not seen in humans except as prolonged impairment of fat absorption.

Vitamin E Megadose Risks

Compared to the other fat-soluble vitamins, vitamin E is relatively nontoxic when taken by mouth; however, supplementation is not recommended unless prescribed for specific needs.

Vitamin K

Major Roles of Vitamin K

Vitamin K aids in the formation of blood-clotting factors and helps maintain normal bone metabolism. The RDA for vitamin K for an adult male is 80 micrograms; for an adult female it is 65 micrograms.

Sources of Vitamin K

The primary source of vitamin K is made by intestinal bacteria. The best dietary source for vitamin K is green leafy vegetables.

Signs of Vitamin K Deficiency

Vitamin K deficiency may cause problems with blood clotting.

In adults, extra vitamin K may be needed by persons on prolonged antibiotic therapy and those with impaired fat absorption, cancer, or kidney disease.

Vitamin K Megadose Risks

Toxic manifestations from excessive intake of vitamin K have not been observed.

WATER-SOLUBLE VITAMINS

In contrast to fat-soluble vitamins **water-soluble vitamins** are not stored in the body, so it is essential that an adequate supply of these vitamins be consumed each day.

Also, water-soluble vitamins are fragile. These vitamins are naturally present in food; however, large portions of these vitamins may be destroyed during food preparation.

The water-soluble vitamins are vitamin C and all of the group referred to as the B-complex vitamins.

Vitamin C

Major Roles of Vitamin C

Vitamin C, also known as **ascorbic acid,** is an antioxidant that also aids in the formation of collagen and is essential for normal wound healing. **Collagen** is a protein substance that holds body cells together.

Vitamin C also helps maintain immunity, capillaries,

bones, and teeth and aids in the absorption of iron. The RDA for vitamin C for adult males and females is 60 milligrams.

Sources of Vitamin C

Citrus fruits, tomatoes, cabbage, cauliflower, melons, strawberries, and dark-green vegetables such as broccoli and brussels sprouts are all good sources of vitamin C.

Signs of Vitamin C Deficiency

A severe deficiency of vitamin C causes **scurvy.** The onset of scurvy is slow and is characterized by capillary bleeding and the weakening of collagenous structures. Other symptoms include wounds that do not heal, degenerating muscles, and brown, rough, dry skin.

Dental signs, which appear later in the disease, include severe gingival enlargement with spontaneous bleeding. After prolonged periodontal involvement, the teeth may loosen and eventually fall out.

Vitamin C Megadose Risks

Vitamin C megadose risks include diarrhea, kidney and bladder stones, and an increased tendency for blood to clot abnormally.

B-Complex Vitamins

Because of their interrelationship, the vitamins that follow are often referred to as a family or as the B-complex vitamins.

Several things happen because of this interrelationship:

- These vitamins are generally found in the same foods.
- They are closely related in the functions they perform.

- No single vitamin in this group is more important than another.
- An inadequate intake of one will impair the utilization of the others. For this reason it is difficult to identify a deficiency disorder that is caused by only one vitamin in the group.
- An excessive intake of one may impair the utilization of the others. For this reason it is difficult to identify a megadose risk that is caused by only one vitamin in the group.

Oral Manifestations of B-Complex Deficiencies

The following is a composite picture of the oral manifestations of a B-complex deficiency. However, it is important to note that other problems may cause many of these same symptoms.

The Lips

There is pallor (paleness), degeneration, and inflammation of the lips and corners of the mouth. As the condition progresses, **cheilosis** may develop. This is characterized by cracks and fissures (deep cracks) along the edges of the lips and at the corners of the mouth. Because of the soreness of the lips, there may be pain upon opening the mouth.

The Tongue

Glossitis, inflammation of the tongue, is characterized by changes in the color and appearance of the tongue. The tongue may become fiery red or purplish red. In some cases the tongue becomes smooth and dry in appearance.

There also may be a burning and tingling sensation of the tongue, and swallowing may be difficult because the tongue is sore.

The Oral Mucosa

The mucous membranes may become inflamed, fiery red, and swollen. There also may be a breakdown of the lining of the buccal mucosa.

There may be excessive salivation because of the soreness of the mouth.

Thiamin

Major Roles of Thiamin

Thiamin, also known as vitamin B_1, releases energy from carbohydrates and aids in the synthesis of important nervous-system chemicals. The RDA for thiamin for an adult male is 1.5 milligrams; for an adult female it is 1.1 milligrams.

Beriberi is a thiamin deficiency disease. In its severe forms it affects the cardiovascular, muscular, and nervous systems.

Sources of Thiamin

Thiamin is found in organ meats (liver, heart, kidney), pork, and enriched and whole-grain products such as cereals, pasta, and bread.

Riboflavin

Major Roles of Riboflavin

Riboflavin, also known as vitamin B_2, helps release energy from carbohydrates and is essential to the functioning of vitamins B_6 and niacin. It also aids in the maintenance of the mucous membranes. The RDA for riboflavin for an adult male is 1.7 milligrams; for an adult female it is 1.3 milligrams.

Ariboflavinosis is a riboflavin deficiency disorder. This is characterized by cheilosis and glossitis in which the tongue takes on a purplish red color.

Sources of Riboflavin

The best animal sources of riboflavin are meats, poultry, fish, and especially dairy products. Grain products naturally contain a relatively low level of riboflavin; however, enriched and fortified cereals, pasta, and bread supply large amounts.

Niacin

Major Roles of Niacin

Niacin, also known as vitamin B_3, **nicotinic acid** and **niacinamide,** acts as a coenzyme in facilitating energy production and tissue respiration in cells. The RDA for niacin for an adult male is 19 milligrams; for an adult female it is 15 milligrams.

Pellagra, caused by a deficiency of niacin, is characterized by the "four D's": diarrhea, dermatitis (skin disorders), dementia (nervous and mental disorders), and, if untreated, death.

Sources of Niacin

Niacin is found in liver, poultry, meat, tuna, eggs, whole-grain and enriched cereals, pasta, and bread. The body also can convert tryptophan into niacin.

Vitamin B_6

Vitamin B_6 comprises three chemically, metabolically, and functionally related forms. These are **pyridoxine, pyridoxal,** and **pyridoxamine.** This vitamin is sometimes identified by these terms.

Major Roles of Vitamin B_6

Vitamin B_6 contributes to the formation of red blood cells and infection-fighting antibodies. It also plays an essential role in the absorption and metabolism of proteins and helps the body use fats. The RDA for vitamin B_6 for an adult male is two milligrams; for an adult female it is 1.6 milligrams.

Excess quantities of vitamin B_6 cause tingling and/or shooting pains in the arms and legs, numbness in the hands and feet, depression, and headaches.

Sources of Vitamin B_6

The richest sources of vitamin B_6 are chicken, fish, kidney, liver, pork, and eggs. Other good sources are unmilled rice, soybeans, oats, whole-wheat products, peanuts, and walnuts. Dairy products and red meats are relatively poor sources.

Folic Acid

Major Roles of Folic Acid

Folic acid, also known as **folate** and **folacin,** acts as a coenzyme in synthesizing genetic material. It also aids in protein metabolism and in the formation of hemoglobin in red blood cells. **Hemoglobin** is the iron-containing portion of the red blood cells.

Recent research indicates that a shortage of folic acid may contribute to birth defects such as **spina bifida** (a birth defect in which the spinal cord is not properly encased in bone) and **anencephaly** (a fatal defect in which part of the brain never develops). An important factor is that this prenatal development occurs during the first two weeks of pregnancy—often before the mother realizes that she is expecting.

The RDA for folic acid for adult males and females is two micrograms.

Sources of Folic Acid

Folic acid sources include leafy-green vegetables, liver, oranges, peanuts, **legumes** (especially dried beans), sunflower seeds, and wheat germ.

Vitamin B$_{12}$

Major Roles of Vitamin B$_{12}$

Vitamin B$_{12}$, also known as **cobalamin,** aids in the formation of red blood cells. It also assists in the building of genetic material and helps the functioning of the nervous system. The RDA for vitamin B$_{12}$ for adult males and females is two micrograms.

Pernicious anemia is caused by a vitamin B_{12} deficiency. This is most likely seen in vegetarians who eat no animal or dairy foods; however, it may also be caused by the body's failure to absorb the vitamin.

Oral manifestations of this disease may be a burning sensation, numbness, or a smooth, bright-red appearance of the tip and margins of the tongue.

Sources of Vitamin B_{12}

Significant sources of vitamin B_{12} include liver, kidney, meat, fish, eggs, dairy products, oysters, and nutritional yeast.

Vitamin B_{12} is not present in any significant amount in plants. Therefore, getting adequate quantities of this nutrient can be a concern for strict vegetarians.

Biotin

Major Roles of Biotin

Biotin aids in the formation of fatty acids and helps release energy from carbohydrates. It is also essential for many enzyme functions. The estimated safe and adequate daily dietary intake of biotin for adults is 30 to 100 milligrams.

Sources of Biotin

Biotin sources include liver, egg yolk, soy flour, and cereals. Fruit and meat are poor sources of biotin. Biotin is also synthesized by microorganisms in the intestinal tract.

Pantothenic Acid

Major Roles of Pantothenic Acid

Pantothenic acid helps in the metabolism of carbohydrates, proteins, and fats. It also aids in the formation of hormones and nerve-regulating substances. The estimated safe and adequate daily dietary intake of pantothenic acid for adults is four to seven milligrams.

Sources of Pantothenic Acid

Pantothenic acid is widely distributed among foods. It is especially abundant in meat, whole-grain cereals, and legumes. It is lost in refined and heavily processed foods.

REVIEW EXERCISES _____

MULTIPLE CHOICE

Circle the correct answer for each question.

1. _____ is the precursor of vitamin A.

   a) Beta carotene
   b) Biotin
   c) Niacin

2. Vitamin _____ assists in the absorption and use of calcium and phosphorus.

   a) C
   b) D
   c) K

3. Cheilosis is an indication of a vitamin _____ deficiency.

   a) B-complex
   b) C
   c) E

4. Citrus fruits and dark-green vegetables are good sources of _____.

   a) niacin
   b) riboflavin
   c) vitamin C

5. A deficiency of folic acid has been linked to _____.

   a) beriberi
   b) rickets
   c) spina bifida

6. A/An _____ is a substance that slows the deterioration of materials through the oxidation process.

   a) antioxidant
   b) coenzyme
   c) oxygen-free radical

7. An excessive intake of one B vitamin _____ make
   up for a shortage of another vitamin in the
   B-complex group.

   a) will
   b) will not

8. _____ -soluble vitamins are not stored in the body,
   so an adequate supply of these vitamins must be
   consumed each day.

   a) Fat
   b) Water

9. The primary source of vitamin _____ is made by
   intestinal bacteria.

   a) B_{12}
   b) E
   c) K

10. Vitamin _____ contributes to the formation of red
    blood cells and infection-fighting antibodies.

    a) B_6
    b) B_{12}
    c) C

SUGGESTED CLASS ACTIVITY

Use the chart that follows to create a list of the primary sources of each vitamin. Circle each of the food sources that you have eaten in the past 24 hours. Based on this information, does it seem that you are getting adequate vitamins from your diet?

Vitamin	Source
Vitamin A	
Vitamin D	
Vitamin E	
Vitamin K	
Vitamin C	
Thiamin (vitamin B_1)	
Riboflavin (vitamin B_2)	
Niacin (vitamin B_2)	
Vitamin B_6	
Folic acid (folacin)	
Vitamin B_{12}	
Biotin	
Pantothenic acid	

CHAPTER 7

MINERALS, TRACE ELEMENTS, AND ELECTROLYTES

OBJECTIVES _____

After studying this chapter, you should be able to:

- describe the functions of minerals in human nutrition.
- describe the functions, sources, signs of deficiency, and megadose risks of these minerals: calcium, phosphorus, magnesium, iron, zinc, iodine, and selenium.
- describe the functions, sources, signs of deficiency, and megadose risks of these trace elements: copper, manganese, fluoride, chromium, and molybdenum.
- describe the functions, sources, signs of deficiency, and megadose risks of these electrolytes: sodium, potassium, and chloride.

THE FUNCTIONS OF MINERALS

Minerals are inorganic substances that are necessary in minute amounts for proper growth, development, and optimal health. Minerals make up only three to four percent of total body weight, but they are essential for maintaining the health and well-being of the individual.

The following are the major functions of minerals in the body.

- Minerals are the components of the bones and teeth that make them rigid and strong.
- Minerals play a part in maintaining the natural muscle and nerve reaction to stimulus.
- Minerals help to maintain the acid-base balance and fluid-electrolyte balance in the body.
- Minerals combine with organic compounds to make up certain hormones found in the body.
- Minerals work together; it is important to maintain a balance to prevent deficiencies.
- One mineral cannot usually be administered without affecting the absorption and metabolism of several others.
- Taking excessive amounts of minerals, in some cases as little as twice the RDA, may be harmful.

Classification of Minerals

Minerals may be classified in several ways. In this chapter, they are divided into three major groups. These groups, summarized in Table 7-1, are minerals, trace elements, and electrolytes.

- The **minerals** include calcium, phosphorus, magnesium, iron, zinc, iodine, and selenium.

Classification of Minerals	
Minerals	Calcium
	Phosphorus
	Magnesium
	Iron
	Zinc
	Iodine
	Selenium
Trace elements	Copper
	Manganese
	Fluoride
	Chromium
	Molybdenum
Electrolytes	Sodium
	Potassium
	Chloride

TABLE 7-1   Classification of Minerals

- The **trace elements,** also known as **microminerals,** are minerals needed by the body in very small amounts. The trace elements include copper, manganese, fluoride, chromium, and molybdenum. Although these inorganic nutrients are required in very small amounts, they play an important role in human nutrition.

- **Electrolytes** are minerals which, when dissolved in solution, form positive and negative ions capable of conducting an electric current. Sodium, potassium, and chloride are the major electrolytes which play an important role in the functioning of the body.

MINERALS

Calcium

Major Roles of Calcium

Calcium is an essential nutrient for growth, maintenance, and reproduction. It is important for building bones and teeth and maintaining bone strength. It is also important for:

- muscle contraction and relaxation (including maintaining a normal heartbeat),
- blood clotting,
- transmission of nerve impulses,
- maintaining cell membranes, and
- the activation of enzyme reactions.

Calcium is the most abundant mineral in the human body. It accounts for about 1.5 to two percent of an adult's total body weight. Of this, 99 percent is in the bones and teeth. The other one percent is found in blood, other body fluids, and various soft tissues.

The RDA for calcium for adult males and females is 800 milligrams.

Sources of Calcium

Milk and milk products, sardines, oysters, canned salmon eaten with bones, dark-green leafy vegetables, citrus fruits, and dried beans and peas supply calcium. Table 7-2 shows the calcium content of popular foods.

Figures on calcium intake may be somewhat misleading since the body does not absorb all the calcium that is consumed. Calcium supplements are often recommended. Table 7-3 summarizes information about the use of these supplements.

Food	Serving (calories)	Calcium (mg)
Broccoli, cooked	1/2 cup (23)	89 mg
Carrot, raw	1 medium (31)	19
Egg, boiled	1 large (79)	28
Milk, skim	1 cup (90)	302
Orange, raw	1 medium (65)	56
Sardines, canned with bones	2 sardines (50)	92
Shake, chocolate*	10 ounces (380)	320

*Fastfood shake. Exact values vary with the brand.

TABLE 7-2 Calcium Content of Popular Foods

Signs of Calcium Deficiency

In children, a severe lack of calcium can produce rickets and distorted bone growth. In adults, too little calcium may contribute to osteoporosis. This is discussed in Chapter 9.

In its effort to maintain a constant level of blood calcium, the body can withdraw some of this mineral from bones if the calcium intake is insufficient.

Calcium Megadose Risks

Calcium megadoses may cause drowsiness, extreme lethargy, and impaired absorption of iron, zinc, and manga-

- So that the body can absorb it, calcium must be accompanied by vitamins C and D.

- The body best absorbs calcium supplements in stages of no more than 600 milligrams at a time. Therefore, for best results, supplements should be taken over the course of a day and preferably after a meal.

- Calcium carbonate, the most common form of supplement, yields 40 percent elemental calcium, which can be absorbed by the body. Therefore, in order to consume 1,000 milligrams of elemental calcium, you would have to take 2,500 milligrams of calcium carbonate.

- If a calcium supplement label lists the contents as "600 mg of calcium carbonate per tablet," it provides 240 mg of calcium that the body can use (40 percent of 600).

- If a calcium supplement label lists the contents as "600 mg of calcium (as calcium carbonate) per tablet," it provides 600 mg of calcium that the body can use.

TABLE 7-3 Facts about Calcium Absorption

nese. Also, megadoses may cause calcium deposits in tissues throughout the body which may look like cancer on X-rays.

Phosphorus

Major Roles of Phosphorus

Phosphorus aids the body in building bones and teeth and releasing energy from carbohydrates, proteins, and fats. Phosphorus is also needed for the formation of genetic material, cell membranes, and many enzymes.

Phosphorus is the second major mineral in the body. Approximately 85 percent of it is found in the skeleton, six percent in the muscles, and nine percent in other tissues. The RDA for phosphorus for adult males and females is 800 milligrams.

Sources of Phosphorus

Phosphorus is found in meat, poultry, fish, eggs, dried beans and peas, milk and milk products. It is also found in processed foods, especially soft drinks.

Signs of Phosphorus Deficiency

Signs of phosphorus deficiency include: weakness, loss of appetite, malaise, and bone pain. Dietary shortages are uncommon, but prolonged use of antacids may cause a deficiency.

Phosphorus Megadose Risks

Distortion of the calcium-to-phosphorus ratio, creating a relative calcium deficiency, may result from phosphorus megadoses.

Magnesium

Major Roles of Magnesium

Magnesium aids bone growth and the manufacture of proteins. It also aids in the release of energy from muscle glycogen and the conduction of nerve impulses to muscles.

The RDA for magnesium for adult males is 350 milligrams; for adult females it is 280 milligrams.

Sources of Magnesium

Leafy green vegetables (eaten raw), nuts (especially almonds and cashews), soybeans, seeds, and whole grains are good magnesium sources.

Signs of Magnesium Deficiency

Signs of magnesium deficiency include: muscle twitching and tremors, irregular heartbeat, insomnia, muscle weakness, and leg and foot cramps.

Deficiency may occur in persons with prolonged diarrhea, kidney disease, diabetes, epilepsy, or alcoholism. Prolonged use of diuretics may also produce a magnesium deficiency.

Magnesium Megadose Risks

Because the calcium-to-magnesium ratio is unbalanced, magnesium megadoses may cause disturbed nervous system function.

Iron

Major Roles of Iron

Iron aids in the formation of hemoglobin in blood and myoglobin in muscles (which supplies oxygen to cells). Iron is also a part of several enzymes and proteins.

The RDA for iron for an adult male is 10 milligrams; for an adult female it is 15 milligrams.

Sources of Iron

Iron is found in liver, kidney, red meats, egg yolk, green leafy vegetables, dried fruits (such as raisins, apricots, and prunes), dried beans and peas, potatoes, blackstrap molasses, and enriched and whole-grain cereals.

Signs of Iron Deficiency

Lack of iron may cause iron deficiency **anemia** with fatigue, weakness, pallor, and shortness of breath. **Anemia,** which takes many forms, is characterized by a reduction in the size or number of red blood cells, the quantity of hemoglobin, or both.

Iron Megadose Risks

Recent studies have linked excess amounts of iron to heart disease. Too much iron may also produce toxic build-up in the liver, pancreas, and heart.

Zinc

Major Roles of Zinc

Zinc is a constituent of about 100 enzymes. Zinc also has a role in cell growth, healing, and the function of the immune system.

The RDA for zinc in an adult male is 15 milligrams; for an adult female it is 12 milligrams.

Sources of Zinc

Sources of zinc include meat, liver, eggs, poultry, seafood, and whole-grain cereals.

Signs of Zinc Deficiency

Signs of zinc deficiency include: delayed wound healing, skin lesions, diminished taste sensation, and a loss of appetite. It may also impact the ability of the immune system to respond.

In children, zinc deficiency may result in failure to grow and mature sexually. Prenatally, too little zinc may cause abnormal brain development.

Zinc Megadose Risks

Megadoses may result in nausea and vomiting, anemia, and bleeding in the stomach. Megadoses may also cause premature birth and stillbirth.

Iodine

Major Roles of Iodine

Iodine is a part of the thyroid hormones. It is also essential for normal reproduction.

The RDA for iodine for adult males and females is 150 micrograms.

Sources of Iodine

Iodine is found in seafood, iodized salt, saltwater fish, seaweed, and sea salt.

Signs of Iodine Deficiency

A lack of iodine, which results in deficient thyroid function, may cause goiter and cretinism.

Simple goiter is a chronic enlargement of the thyroid gland caused by a lack of dietary iodine. (There are also many other types of goiter.) In the past this form of goiter was found in areas where the dietary intake of iodine was less than adequate, for example, inland areas where the residents did not have access to seafood, a good source of iodine. Since table salt is now routinely iodized, i.e. has iodine added to it, this form of simple goiter is no longer a common problem.

Cretinism, which appears during the first years of life, is characterized by stunted body growth and mental development. It may result from an inadequate maternal intake of iodine during pregnancy.

Iodine Megadose Risks

Iodine megadoses are not known to be a problem, but they could cause iodine poisoning or sensitivity reaction.

Selenium

Major Roles of Selenium

Selenium is an antioxidant, preventing the breakdown of fats and other body chemicals. It also interacts with vitamin E.

The RDA for selenium for an adult male is 70 micrograms; for an adult female it is 55 micrograms.

Sources of Selenium

Selenium is found in seafood, whole-grain cereals, meat, egg yolk, chicken, milk, and garlic.

Signs of Selenium Deficiency

The effects of selenium deficiency are not known in human beings. In animals it causes degeneration of the pancreas.

Selenium Megadose Risks

In animals megadoses may produce "blind staggers"—stiffness, lameness, hair loss, blindness, and death.

TRACE ELEMENTS

Copper

Major Roles of Copper

Copper aids in the formation of red blood cells. It is also part of several respiratory enzymes.

The estimated safe and adequate daily dietary intake of copper for healthy adults is 1.5 to three milligrams.

Sources of Copper

Sources of copper include: oysters, nuts, cocoa powder, beef and pork liver, kidney, dried beans, and corn oil margarine.

Signs of Copper Deficiency

In animals, too little copper may cause anemia, faulty development of bone and nerve tissue, loss of elasticity in tendons and major arteries, and abnormal structure and pigmentation of hair.

Copper Megadose Risks

Megadose risks include violent vomiting and diarrhea. Cooking acid foods in unlined copper pans may lead to a toxic accumulation of copper.

Manganese

Major Roles of Manganese

Manganese is needed for functioning of the central nervous system, normal bone structure, and reproduction. Manganese is also a component of certain important enzymes.

The estimated safe and adequate daily dietary intake of manganese for healthy adults is two to five milligrams.

Sources of Manganese

Sources of manganese include nuts, whole grains, vegetables and fruits, tea, instant coffee, and cocoa powder.

Signs of Manganese Deficiency

The effects of manganese deficiency are not known in human beings. In animals it causes poor reproduction, retarded growth, birth defects, and abnormal bone development.

Manganese Megadose Risks

Too much manganese may cause a mask-like facial expression, slurred speech, involuntary laughing, spastic gait, and hand tremors.

Fluoride

Major Roles Of Fluoride

Fluoride aids in the formation of strong decay-resistant teeth. Because it plays such an important role in preventive dentistry, fluoride is discussed further in Chapter 11.

The estimated safe and adequate daily dietary intake of fluoride for a healthy adult is 1.5 to four milligrams.

Sources of Fluoride

Fluoride may occur naturally in water or be added to the water supply. It is also found in foods prepared with water containing fluoride.

Signs of Fluoride Deficiency

Lack of fluoride may contribute to excessive dental decay.

Fluoride Megadose Risks

The fluoride megadose risks include fluorosis and, in extreme cases, poisoning.

Chromium

Major Roles Of Chromium

Chromium helps glucose metabolism. It may also help lower elevated blood sugars in diabetics.

The estimated safe and adequate daily dietary intake of chromium for a healthy adult is 50 to 200 micrograms.

Sources of Chromium

Sources of chromium include meat, cheese, whole-grain breads and cereals, dried beans, peanuts, and brewer's yeast.

Signs of Chromium Deficiency

Chromium deficiency may possibly cause abnormal sugar metabolism (chemical diabetes) and maturity-onset diabetes.

Chromium Megadose Risks

There are no known megadose risks.

Molybdenum

Major Roles Of Molybdenum

Molybdenum mobilizes iron from liver reserves. It oxidizes fats and is an important component of several enzyme systems.

The estimated safe and adequate daily dietary intake of molybdenum for a healthy adult is 75 to 250 micrograms.

Sources of Molybdenum

Sources of molybdenum include dried peas and beans, cereal grains, liver, kidney, and dark-green leafy vegetables.

Signs of Molybdenum Deficiency

Risks of molybdenum deficiency are not known in human beings. In animals, it may result in decreased weight gain and shortened life span.

Molybdenum Megadose Risks

Molybdenum megadose risks are a gout-like syndrome and the loss of copper.

ELECTROLYTES

Potassium

Major Roles of Potassium

Potassium is needed for muscle contraction and maintenance of the fluid and electrolyte balance in cells. It also aids in the transmission of nerve impulses and the release of energy from carbohydrates, proteins, and fat.

Only a minimum daily requirement has been established for potassium. This is 1,600 to 2,000 milligrams per day; however, actual needs are probably much higher.

Sources of Potassium

Potassium is found in orange juice, bananas, fresh fruits, meats, bran, peanut butter, dried beans and peas, potatoes, coffee, tea, and cocoa.

Signs of Potassium Deficiency

A potassium deficiency may cause abnormal heart rhythm, muscular weakness, lethargy, and kidney and lung failure.

A deficiency may occur among heavy laborers and athletes who work hard in heat. It may also occur in persons with prolonged diarrhea or individuals who are taking diuretics and purgatives (laxatives). **Diuretics** are drugs that increase the production of urine and reduce the volume of fluid in the body.

Potassium Megadose Risks

Excessive potassium in the blood may cause muscular paralysis and abnormal heart rhythm.

Sodium

Major Roles of Sodium

Sodium, working with chloride, helps regulate the balance of water in the body. It also has a role in the functioning of nerves and muscles. In addition, it aids in the passage of substances in and out of cells.

The estimated safe and adequate daily dietary intake of sodium for healthy persons is five milligrams.

Sources of Sodium

Sodium is found in table salt (sodium chloride); however, only about 10 percent of the dietary intake comes from table salt added to food. The major source of sodium is prepared foods.

Signs of Sodium Deficiency

Sodium depletion may be caused by heavy and persistent sweating or where there is injury, chronic diarrhea, or renal disease that produces an inability to retain sodium.

The symptoms of sodium deficiency include severe muscle cramps, extreme weakness, nausea, and diarrhea.

Sodium Megadose Risks

As long as the body's water needs are met, acute toxicity from excessive dietary sodium is not a major risk because the kidneys can excrete the excess.

Excessive dietary sodium has been implicated in high blood pressure, heart disease, and stroke.

Chloride

Major Roles of Chloride

Chloride helps to maintain the acid-base and the fluid balance of the body. It also activates salivary amylase (the enzyme in saliva) and serves as part of stomach acid.

The estimated safe and adequate daily dietary intake of chloride for healthy persons is 750 milligrams.

Sources of Chloride

Chloride is found in table salt and other naturally occurring salts.

Signs of Chloride Deficiency

A lack of chloride can cause a disturbed acid-base balance in body fluids. This occurs very rarely.

Chloride Megadose Risks

Megadoses of chloride can bring about a disturbed acid-base balance.

REVIEW EXERCISES _____

MULTIPLE CHOICE

Circle the correct answer for each question.

1. Apricots and prunes are good sources of _____.

   a) calcium
   b) iron
   c) magnesium

2. A/An _____ is a mineral which is needed by the body in very small amounts.

   a) electrolyte
   b) trace mineral

3. _____ is the most abundant mineral in the human body.

   a) Calcium
   b) Iron
   c) Phosphorus

4. Signs of a _____ deficiency include delayed wound healing.

   a) chromium
   b) selenium
   c) zinc

5. _____, working with chloride, helps regulate the balance of water in the body.

   a) Fluoride
   b) Potassium
   c) Sodium

6. _____ consumption must be accompanied by vitamins A and D.

   a) Calcium
   b) Iodine
   c) Molybdenum

7. _____, which is found abundantly in red meats, aids in the formation of hemoglobin in the blood.

   a) Copper
   b) Iodine
   c) Iron

8. _____ is/are naturally occurring in table salt.

   a) Chloride
   b) Sodium
   c) A and B

9. _____, which is found in nuts, tea, and instant coffee, is a trace element that is needed for functioning of the central nervous system.

   a) Chromium
   b) Manganese
   c) Molybdenum

10. Potassium is a/an _____.

   a) electrolyte
   b) micromineral
   c) trace element

SUGGESTED CLASS ACTIVITY

Use the chart that follows to create a list of the major minerals and the primary sources of each. Circle each of the food sources that you have eaten in the past 24 hours. Based on this information, does it seem that you are getting adequate minerals from your diet?

Mineral	Source
Calcium	
Iodine	
Iron	
Magnesium	
Phosphorus	
Selenium	
Zinc	

SUGGESTED CLASS DISCUSSION

Look at Table 7-2. Discuss which of these foods would best enable you to have an adequate dietary calcium intake without consuming excessive calories.

CHAPTER 8

DIETARY GUIDELINES

OBJECTIVES _____

After studying this chapter, you should be able to:

- list the seven key points in the Dietary Guidelines for Americans.
- describe the five food groups in terms of the foods included in each and the number of recommended servings per day from each group.
- calculate the recommended maximum number of grams of fat in relation to daily caloric intake.
- explain how the Food Guide Pyramid is used as an aid in selecting a healthy diet.
- identify the two agencies that regulate food labeling requirements.
- state the information required on food labels regarding carbohydrates.
- describe how fats are listed on a food label.

OVERVIEW

In the previous chapters you learned about the nutrients and how the body utilizes them. In this chapter you will learn how to select the foods that will provide these nutrients in the appropriate balance to help keep your body healthy.

This chapter focuses on the dietary choices for a healthy individual. In Chapter 9 you will learn about individuals with special dietary needs.

DIETARY GUIDELINES FOR AMERICANS

In 1990 the United States Department of Agriculture (USDA) and the Department of Health and Human Services (HHS) issued *Dietary Guidelines for Americans.* The purpose of these guidelines is to help Americans be healthier by modifying their dietary and lifestyle choices.

These guidelines are advice for healthy individuals aged two years and over. They *are not* designed for younger children and infants whose dietary needs differ. These special needs are discussed in Chapter 9.

The guidelines emphasize the following key points:

- Eat a variety of foods.
- Maintain healthy weight.
- Choose a diet low in fat, saturated fat, and cholesterol.
- Choose a diet with plenty of vegetables, fruits, and grain products.
- Use sugars in moderation.
- Use salt and sodium in moderation.
- If you drink alcoholic beverages, do so in moderation.

Eat a Variety of Foods

As you learned in the previous chapters, nutrients come from a variety of foods. Dietary choices should not be limited to a few highly fortified foods or supplements. Many foods are a good source of several nutrients. For example, vegetables and fruits are important for vitamins A and C, folic acid, minerals, and fiber. However, no single food can supply all nutrients in the amounts needed.

One way to assure variety is to choose foods each day from the major food groups. The *Food Guide Pyramid,* which is discussed later in this chapter, is an aid to selecting foods in the appropriate proportions.

Maintain Healthy Weight

If you are too fat or too thin, your chances of developing health problems are increased. Table 8-1 shows a suggested range of weights for adults. In this table the higher weights in the ranges generally apply to men who tend to have more muscle and bone. The lower weights more often apply to women, who have less muscle and bone.

Although this table suggests a recommended weight range, research indicates that a "healthy" weight depends on how much of your weight is fat, where the fat is located in your body, and whether you have weight-related medical problems.

Choose a Diet Low in Fat, Saturated Fat, and Cholesterol

The recommended goal is to have only 30 percent of your daily caloric intake come from all sources of fats—preferably

Height	Weight in Pounds (19 to 34 years)	Weight in Pounds (35 years and over)
5'0"	97-128	108-138
5'1"	101-132	111-143
5'2"	104-137	115-148
5'3"	107-141	119-152
5'4"	111-146	122-157
5'5"	114-150	126-162
5'6"	118-155	130-167
5'7"	121-160	134-172
5'8"	125-164	138-178
5'9"	125-164	138-178
5'10"	132-174	146-188
5'11"	136-179	151-194
6'0"	140-184	155-199
6'1"	144-189	159-205
6'2"	148-195	164-210
6'3"	152-200	168-210
6'4"	156-205	173-222
6'5"	160-211	177-228
6'6"	164-216	182-234

Source: Nutrition and Your Health: Dietary Guidelines for Americans. 3rd edition. U.S. Department of Agriculture: U.S. Department of Health and Human Services, 1990.

TABLE 8-1 Suggested Range of Weights for Adults

from unsaturated fats. Some health authorities feel that it would be even better if the total fat intake were limited to 25 percent or less of calories.

The American Heart Association recommends that saturated fatty acid intake should be less than 10 percent of calories and that cholesterol intake should be no more than 300 milligrams per day. They also recommend that polyunsaturated fatty acid intake should be less than 10 percent of calories and that monounsaturated fatty acids make up the rest of the total fat intake.

Calculating Fat Percentage

The following formula can be used to calculate the maximum amount of fat per day in proportion to your caloric intake.

Step 1: Multiply 30 percent by the number of calories per day. This equals the maximum desirable number of calories from fat.

Step 2: Divide the number of calories by nine (there are nine calories per gram of fat). This equals the maximum number of grams per day for all fat sources.

Here is an example showing how these calculations work.

- 30 percent × 2,000 calories per day = 600 calories from fat.
- Divide 600 by nine calories per gram of fat = 66.66.
- This equals approximately 67 grams of total fat allowable per day.

Table 8-2 shows examples of how these calculations work for a given number of calories. Table 8-3 illustrates a short cut for performing these calculations.

Calories	Grams of fat (30% limit)
1,200	40
1,500	50
2,000	67
2,500	83
3,000	100

TABLE 8-2   Allowable Grams of Fat

Short Cut for Calculating Grams of Fat per Day
To estimate your desirable fat limit in grams of fat per day, divide your ideal weight in half. If your ideal weight is 120 pounds, your desirable limit is 60 grams of fat.

TABLE 8-3   Calculating Grams of Fat per Day

Choose a Diet with Plenty of Vegetables, Fruits, and Grain Products

Vegetables, fruits, and grain products are an important part of a varied diet. They provide complex carbohydrates, dietary fiber, and other nutrients and are generally low in fat.

Use Sugars in Moderation

Sugars and many foods that contain them in large amounts supply calories but are limited in nutrients.

Use Salt and Sodium in Moderation

Most Americans eat more salt and sodium than they need. About one-third of this salt comes from the salt shaker; the balance comes from foods and beverages which have salt added in processing.

The National Heart, Lung, and Blood Institute recommends that people with high blood pressure limit sodium intake to 2,500 milligrams a day. That is about 1 1/4 teaspoon of salt.

If You Drink Alcoholic Beverages, Do So in Moderation

Alcoholic beverages supply calories but little or no nutrients. For this and the reasons listed below, if adults choose to drink, they should have no more than one to two drinks per day.

- Each gram of alcoholic beverage contains seven calories. (These are empty calories with no nutrient value.)
- Drinking alcoholic beverages has no proven net health benefits.
- Drinking alcoholic beverages is linked to many health problems and is the cause of many accidents.
- Drinking alcoholic beverages can lead to addiction.
- Women who are pregnant or trying to conceive should *not* drink alcoholic beverages.

THE FOOD GUIDE PYRAMID

The **Food Guide Pyramid,** which was introduced in 1992, is the visual companion to the written Dietary Guidelines for Americans (Fig. 8-1). The Pyramid emphasizes eating a variety of foods in relative proportions to get the nutri-

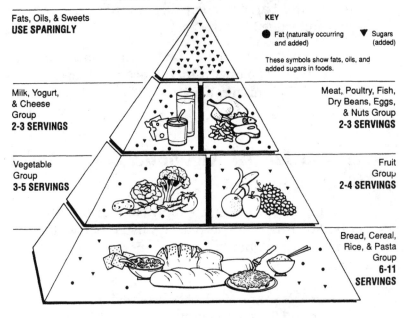

FIGURE 8-1 The Food Pyramid is a visual guide to healthier living. (*Courtesy U.S. Department of Agriculture.*)

ents you need and at the same time the right amount of calories to maintain a healthy weight.

Food Groups

In the *Food Guide Pyramid* the familiar "four food groups" that we learned as children have been replaced by five food groups (Fig. 8-2).

Information about these groups is summarized in Table 8-4. The following are additional important facts about these groups:

- Each of the food groups provides some, but not all, of the nutrients needed daily.
- Foods in one group cannot replace those in another.
- Each food group is needed for good health.
- The key is to eat proportional amounts from each group as demonstrated by the Pyramid.
- A recommended range of servings for each food group is included. Individuals with lower caloric needs should eat the fewer number of servings indicated at the lower end of the range.
- Pay close attention to the recommended serving size. Although many servings are recommended of some foods, the portion sizes are small.

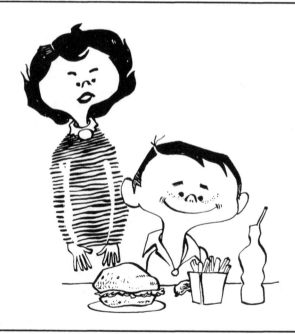

FIGURE 8-2 "No, Jimmy, a hamburger, catsup, fries, a pickle, and a coke are not the five food groups."

Food Group	Suggested Daily Servings	Serving Size
Bread, Cereal, Rice, and Pasta Group	6 to 11	1 slice of bread 1/2 bun, bagel, or english muffin 1 oz. ready-to-eat cereal 1/2 cup cooked cereal 1/2 cup cooked pasta, rice, or grits
Vegetable Group	3 to 5	1/2 cup cooked vegetable 1/2 cup chopped raw vegetable 1 cup leafy raw vegetable
Fruit Group	2 to 4	whole piece of fruit 1/2 cup juice 1/4 melon 1/2 grapefruit 1/2 cup cooked or canned fruit 1/4 cup dried fruit
Milk, Yogurt, and Cheese Group	2 to 3 Children teens, and women up to 25 yrs of age should have 3 to 4 servings per day.	1 cup lowfat or skim milk 1 cup lowfat yogurt 1 1/2 oz. lowfat cheese
Meat, Poultry, Fish, Dried	2 to 3	2-3 oz. cooked lean meat, fish, or

Food Group	Suggested Daily Servings	Serving Size
Beans, Eggs, and Nuts Group		poultry 2 eggs 1 cup cooked dried beans or peas 2 tablespoons peanut butter
Fats, Oils, and Sweets Group	No recommended daily servings. Use sparingly.	Spreads, oils, salad dressings, candy, many refined carbohydrates, etc.

TABLE 8-4   Food Group Information from the Food Pyramid

At the Base of the Pyramid

These are foods from plant sources:

- In the *Bread, Cereal, Rice, and Pasta Group,* six to 11 servings are recommended daily. (Serving sizes: one slice of bread; one oz. ready-to-eat cereal; 1/2 cup cooked cereal, 1/2 cup pasta, rice, or grits.)

On the Second Level

These are foods from plant sources:

- In the *Vegetable Group,* three to five servings are recommended daily. (Serving sizes: 1/2 cup cooked vegetable, 1/2 cup chopped raw vegetable, one cup leafy raw vegetable.)
- In the *Fruit Group,* two to four servings are recom-

mended daily. (Serving sizes: whole piece of fruit, 1/2 cup juice, 1/4 melon, 1/2 grapefruit, 1/2 cup cooked or canned fruit, 1/4 cup dried fruit.)

On the Third Level

These are mostly foods from animal sources (with the exception of nuts and dried beans).

- In the *Milk, Yogurt, and Cheese Group*, two to three servings are recommended daily. Children, teens, and women up to 25 years of age should have three to four servings per day. (Serving sizes: one cup skim or one percent lowfat milk, one cup lowfat yogurt, 1 1/2 oz. lowfat cheese.)
- In the *Meat, Poultry, Fish, Dried Beans, Eggs, and Nuts Group*, two to three servings are recommended daily. (Serving sizes: two to three oz. cooked lean meat, fish, or poultry; two eggs; one cup cooked dried beans or peas; two tablespoons peanut butter. [The serving size for a piece of meat is about the size of a deck of playing cards].)

At the Tip of the Pyramid

These are foods that provide calories but little else nutritionally. These should be used sparingly:

- The *Fats, Oils, and Sweets Group* should be used sparingly; there are no recommended daily servings for this group. In addition to appearing in this group, the symbols for fat and sugars are also shown in the other groups. This serves as a reminder that some food choices in other groups can also be high in fat or added sugars.

FOOD LABELING INFORMATION

Food labels are an important source of information regarding the nutrients contained in a given food. Carefully reading these labels is very helpful in planning a healthy diet.

Labeling requirements are controlled by two government agencies. They are the United States Department of Agriculture (USDA) for meat, poultry, and eggs and the Federal Food and Drug Administration (FDA) for most other food products.

Nutrition Labeling and Education Act (NLEA)

The **1990 Nutrition Labeling and Education Act (NLEA)** mandates sweeping changes in the nutrition information listed on food packages, effective in 1994. Figure 8-3 illustrates the information included on a macaroni and cheese label that meets these new requirements.

This law makes nutritional information labeling mandatory for most foods under FDA jurisdiction and focuses on making it consistent with current knowledge of diet and health.

Labels include the following information:

- *Serving size* and *servings per container.* Serving size has been standardized to represent a reasonable quantity used by an adult.
- *Calories* per serving and the *calories from fat.*
- *Protein* is shown as the number of grams per serving.
- *Total carbohydrate* is listed in grams and as the percentage of the daily value. The amount of *sugar* and *dietary fiber* are listed in grams.
- *Sodium* is listed in grams and as the percentage of the daily value.

NUTRITION FACTS

Serving Size	1-1/4 cup (1 ounce)
Servings per Container	15
Calories 175	Calories from fat 27

Amount per serving	% Daily Value *
Total Fat 3 g	5%
Saturated Fat 0g	0%
Cholesterol 0g	0%
Sodium 330 mg	14%
Total Carbohydrate 30g	10%
Sugars 7 g	
Dietary Fiber 2.5g	10%
Protein 15g	

Vitamin A 30%, Vitamin C 25%, Calcium 20%, Iron 45%

* Percents (%) of a Daily Value are based on a 2,000 diet. Your Daily Values may vary high or lower depending on your calorie needs:

Nutrient		2,000 Calories	2,500 Calories
Total Fat	less than	65g	80g
Sat Fat	less than	20g	25g
Cholesterol	less than	300mg	300mg
Sodium	less than	2,400mg	2,400mg
Total Carbohydrate		300g	375g
Fiber		25g	30g

1g Fat = 9 calories
1g Carbohydrate = 4 calories
1g Protein = 4 calories

FIGURE 8-3 A hypothetical label for cereal and skim milk that meets new labeling requirements.

- *Total fat* and *saturated fat* are listed in grams.
- *Cholesterol* is listed in milligrams. All are also listed as the percentage of the daily value.

Information regarding the portion of daily requirements provided in each serving is based on a 2,000 calorie diet, which applies to most women, and a 2,500 diet, which is applicable to most men.

DIET DIARY

A diet diary is a simple tool that is used in order to record information that evaluates how well you are doing in meeting your nutritional needs (Fig. 8-4).

In its simplest form a diet diary is just a listing of all foods eaten within a 24-hour period. However, it is important to include certain details. These include:

- What time did you eat? Was this part of a meal, or was it a snack?
- What did you eat (name each food)?
- How was each food prepared?
- What serving size did you have of each food?
- Be sure to list the "extras" such as butter, jam, or salad dressing.
- Don't forget to list all snacks and munchies.

Suggested art for Figure 8-4 Diet Diary

Time	Food eaten and quantity (when applicable, note how prepared)
7 A.M.	6 oz orange juice
	1 oz corn flakes with 4 oz skim milk
	1 slice whole wheat toast with butter and jam
	2 cups of coffee with sugar and cream
10 A.M.	1 jelly donut
	1 cup coffee with sugar and cream
12:30	Fast Food Double cheeseburger with bacon
	chocolate shake
	fries
4: P.M.	candy bar
6:30	1/2 fried chicken
	mashed potatoes with gravy
	1/2 c. boiled string beans
	1 slice apple pie with ice cream
	diet coke
10: P.M.	8 oz skim milk
	4 oreo cookies

FIGURE 8-4   A sample diet diary page.

REVIEW EXERCISES _____

MULTIPLE CHOICE

Circle the correct answer for each question.

1. From the bread, cereal, rice, and pasta group, _____ servings are suggested daily.

   a) two to three
   b) six to 11
   c) eight to 15

2. The serving size for a piece of lean meat is _____ ounces.

   a) two to three
   b) three to five
   c) five to eight

3. A serving of whole milk contains nine grams of fat. This means that there are _____ calories from fat in a serving of whole milk.

   a) 36
   b) 63
   c) 81

4. A serving of whole milk contains _____ than the recommended proportion of dietary fat (30%).

   a) less
   b) more

5. If you had a sandwich for lunch (made with two pieces of bread), you would have eaten _____ serving(s) of bread.

   a) one
   b) 1 1/2
   c) two

6. Labeling requirements for meat, poultry, and eggs are mandated by the _____.

   a) Federal Food and Drug Administration (FDA)
   b) United States Department of Agriculture (USDA)

7. For foods listed at the tip of the *Food Pyramid* (fats and sugars), _____ servings are recommended daily.

   a) zero
   b) one to two
   c) three to four

8. If you consume 1,200 calories per day, your fat intake should be limited to no more than _____ grams of fat per day.

   a) 30
   b) 40
   c) 80

9. On a food label, dietary fiber is listed _____.

   a) as a percentage of the daily requirement
   b) in grams
   c) a and b

10. Food labels are required to indicate the amount of total fat listed in milligrams and _____.

    a) cholesterol listed in milligrams
    b) saturated fat listed in grams
    c) a and b

SUGGESTED CLASS ACTIVITY

Keep a diet diary for at least one day. Transfer information from your diet diary to the table below to see how well you did in meeting the guidelines.

- Pay close attention to serving sizes.
- For complex foods such as a chicken pot pie, try to break them down into components: meat (chicken), pastry (bread), and vegetables.
- Place foods that don't fit in any category such as candy or soda pop in the last group.

In class, be prepared to discuss how well you did with this experience.

- Was it difficult to keep track of what you ate?
- Did you consume more "servings" than expected in some groups?
- Was it hard to determine which groups some foods belonged in?
- Did you have a lot of foods in the last category?
- How do you feel about how well you did in meeting your daily requirements?

Food Group	Foods Eaten
Bread, Cereal, Rice, and Pasta Group (6 to 11 servings)	
Vegetable Group (3 to 5 servings)	
Fruit Group (2 to 4 servings)	
Milk, Yogurt, and Cheese Group (2 to 3 servings)	
Meat, Poultry, Fish, Dried Beans, Eggs, and Nuts Group (2 to 3 servings)	
Fats, Oils, and Sweets Group (Also "other")	

CHAPTER 9

SPECIAL NUTRITIONAL NEEDS

OBJECTIVES

After studying this chapter, you should be able to:

- state why it is important to seek medical care early in pregnancy.
- describe the role of the mother's dental health on the developing baby.
- describe the steps to be taken to avoid baby bottle syndrome.
- state why infants and young children should not be put on a low-fat diet.
- state the role of sealants in preventive dentistry.
- describe the dental implications of bulimia nervosa.
- state the desirable serum cholesterol level and differentiate between low-density lipoproteins and high-ensity lipoproteins.
- state the blood pressure readings for adults under 40 and over 40 that indicate hypertension.
- list at least five factors that may influence an older person's nutritional status.
- describe the three primary steps to prevent osteoporosis.

OVERVIEW OF SPECIAL NEEDS

In Chapter 8 we looked at guidelines for the general population. In this chapter we will look at the special needs of different age groups. In addition, we will discuss disorders that are related because of their nutritional, dietary, and/or dental implications.

PRENATAL AND PREGNANCY NEEDS

The nutritional status of the mother before and during pregnancy has an important influence on the health of her developing baby. Nutritional imbalances from the very earliest stages of development are important because they have a negative impact on prenatal growth and development. They also may impair later developmental events.

Prenatal Dental Development

Tooth formation begins as early as the sixth week of the baby's development. Calcification (hardening) of the primary teeth begins at four months. Formation, but not calcification, of many of the permanent teeth has already started when the baby is born.

In order to develop healthy bones and teeth, the unborn child must receive from the mother an adequate supply of appropriate nutrients. Calcium and phosphorus are particularly important for dental development.

Maternal Care

The best way to prevent difficulties during pregnancy is to ensure excellent maternal nutrition and health prior to conception and throughout the pregnancy. This is one of many reasons why it is extremely important that the mother receive medical guidance beginning in the very early stages of her pregnancy.

Dental Care

In order to prevent the pain of a toothache or soreness in the mouth that might prevent proper eating, the mother should also receive regular dental care throughout her pregnancy.

The old saying that "the mother will lose a tooth for every child" implies that during each pregnancy the mother will have a tooth extracted because of decay and pain. This is based on the false assumption that the developing baby draws calcium from the mother's teeth. When the mother's diet is deficient in calcium her body may try to compensate for this lack by drawing some calcium from her bones; however, her teeth will not be affected.

When the mother's calcium levels aren't sufficient to meet the needs of the mother and baby, both may suffer because of the deficiency.

INFANCY

This stage of life, between birth and approximately two years of age, is second only to the prenatal stage when it comes to rapidness of body development. Nutritional deficiencies and excesses during infancy can have a negative impact on growth and development throughout an individual's entire life.

Although there is an emphasis on maintaining a low-fat diet for the general public, this does *not* hold true for infants and very young children. At this age they need more fats and cholesterol than at any other time in life. For this reason, unless under medical supervision, a very young child should not be put on a low-fat diet such as giving him only skim milk.

Calcification of the crowns of the permanent teeth begins at birth. With the exception of the third molars, the crowns of permanent teeth have all calcified before eight years of age. The third molars, which do not erupt until the late teens, are usually calcified by age 16.

Baby-Bottle Syndrome (BBS)

The use of the baby bottle as a pacifier, either at night or during the day, is one of the major reasons for a distinct pattern of rapid tooth decay in young children known as **baby-bottle syndrome (BBS).** Since the effects of BBS may not appear until two or three years after the child has given up the baby bottle, prevention starting at birth is extremely important.

Parents should be cautioned to avoid:

- putting flavored milk, juice, soda, or any sweetened substance in the baby bottle. (These cariogenic sweets may encourage dental decay.)
- dipping the bottle nipple or pacifier in honey before giving it to the baby. (The amount of time each day that a child spends sucking on the sweetened bottle is a contributing factor to BBS.)
- putting the child down to sleep with a bottle containing a sweetened substance. (The sweetened residue left on the baby's teeth during sleep also contributes to the problem.)

THE PRESCHOOL CHILD

During the second and third years of life enthusiasm for eating is often notably less than during infancy. The reasons for this apparent decrease in appetite are not completely understood.

One reason may be that the growth rate has decreased, and therefore less energy is needed. Whatever the reason, decreased food intake is so common during this period that it may be considered a characteristic of normal children.

Although many children are picky eaters at this stage, their nutrition is extremely important. Parents should be encouraged to work with the child to make sure that the food eaten meets the child's nutritional needs. It is at this age that children are beginning to develop the food preferences and eating patterns that they will follow throughout life. Parental guidance in food selection and in avoiding frequent sugary and fatty snacks is particularly important.

Dental Caries

Dental caries, commonly known as **decay,** is the destruction of tooth structure. This is caused by the repeated acid attacks on the enamel caused by plaque. The role of plaque is explained in Chapter 12.

Once decay has progressed through the enamel it may travel quickly through the dentin and into the pulp of the tooth. When a tooth has decayed to this extent, it cannot repair itself, and a restoration must be placed.

Sealants

In addition to the preventive measures discussed in this book, **sealants** are an important measure to protect the chewing surfaces of the primary and permanent teeth against decay.

The chewing surfaces of the teeth are formed with deep grooves called **fissures.** Where two fissures cross, they form a **pit.** Because these areas are narrow and deep they are difficult, if not impossible, to clean with a toothbrush. Soon after the tooth has erupted the dentist may place a pit and fissure sealant to seal and protect these areas from decay.

THE SCHOOL-AGE CHILD

Throughout this period the child continues to need a diet that meets his nutritional requirements. Also during this period, lifetime eating patterns are still being established.

In addition to meeting nutritional needs, food has important social, emotional, and psychological implications. The child is having experiences concerning foods that will greatly influence future eating habits. For example:

- favorite childhood foods often remain favorites throughout life.
- foods provided when the child was sick may continue to be considered by the adult as "comfort food" and be particularly desired when the adult is ill or upset.
- the child who is always rewarded with candy and sweets may continue to regard these foods as rewards and make them an important part of life, even after becoming an adult.

Since school-age children have not yet developed the knowledge and experience to make proper food choices entirely by themselves, strong nutritional guidance by well-qualified adults is needed throughout childhood. It is also important at this age that the child begin to learn the essentials of good nutrition and how to select good foods for himself (Fig. 9-1).

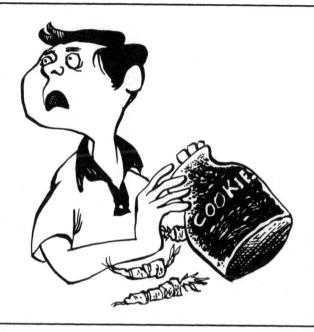

FIGURE 9-1 "Hey—who put carrots in the cookie jar?"

ADOLESCENCE

Adolescence is a period of very rapid physical growth and development, second only to infancy. The adolescent growth spurt may contribute anywhere between 15 to 25 percent of the adult height.

Adolescence is also a period of intense change and stress. During this stage, nutritional and energy needs are greatly accelerated. For these reasons it is particularly important that the diet of the teenager meet his or her nutritional needs, including providing energy from appropriate sources.

Teenagers still need guidance in making dietary choices, but they are not likely to accept it from their parents. Instead, their food habits and choices are greatly influenced by those of their peers, and snacking is an increasingly common lifestyle choice for them (Fig. 9-2).

Nutritional advice for this age group should focus on meeting nutritional needs through a balanced diet. It should stress the importance of avoiding fad diets and begin to emphasize the dietary guidelines described in Chapter 8.

Anorexia Nervosa

Anorexia nervosa is an illness usually occurring in girls shortly after puberty or later in adolescence. It is characterized by excessive self-imposed weight loss and a distorted attitude toward eating and body weight.

Extreme weight loss from anorexia causes a wide range of serious medical complications. These include a failure to develop normally, **amenorrhea** (lack of menstruation), muscular weakness, electrolyte imbalances which may cause sudden death, as well as chronic cardiac (heart) disorders, and renal (kidney) impairment.

Treatment of anorexia nervosa involves physiological means to help the patient gain necessary weight and psychological help to overcome the cause of the disorder.

Some of the chronically ill patients with anorexia nervosa also develop **bulimia nervosa.** They combine a pattern of fasting with binge eating. **Binge eating** is the rapid consumption of large amounts of food in a short period of time.

Bulimia Nervosa

Bulimia nervosa is characterized by recurrent episodes of binge eating followed by "purging"—getting rid of the food which was eaten. Purging includes self-induced vomiting as well as the use of laxatives or diuretics.

This behavior, which occurs almost exclusively in young

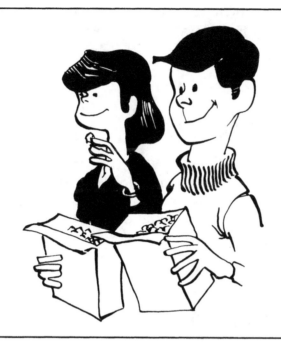

FIGURE 9-2 Popcorn is a healthy and noncariogenic snack food.

women, is associated with serious health consequences. These include electrolyte imbalances which may cause heart failure.

Dental Implications

Bulimia nervosa also has serious dental complications. During vomiting, the tooth surfaces are exposed to highly acidic contents of the stomach. These acids etch and weaken the enamel surfaces of the teeth. Also, brushing the teeth after vomiting seems to further damage the enamel.

Until the condition is under control, the dentist may instruct the patient to rinse her mouth with an alkaline solution instead of brushing immediately after vomiting.

Treatment of bulimia nervosa usually includes psychological and behavioral help to overcome the problem.

ADULTHOOD

Good nutrition's most significant role during youth and middle age is the prevention of those diseases that will ultimately appear as serious disabilities among the aged. Preventive nutrition for aging should begin before birth and continue through all the stages of life.

Bone Formation

From birth to about age 18 or 20, the bones are in a phase of active growth. Active growth is characterized by an increase in bone length and width. However, peak bone mass is probably not attained before age 25.

Although bone growth and shaping of the growing skeleton cease at maturity, adult bone is constantly being remodeled. It is this bone remodeling that makes orthodontic treatment possible.

Remodeling, a continuous maintenance or repair process, is the result of the resorption (loss) of existing bone and the deposition (growth) of new bone to replace that which was removed.

Between ages 30 and 40, resorption of existing bone begins to exceed formation of new bone, resulting in a net loss of bone. Bone loss occurs in both men and women, and once begun, continues throughout the rest of life. **Osteoporosis,** the result of excessive bone loss, is discussed later in this chapter.

Serum Cholesterol

Cholesterol is a complex, fat-related compound found in practically all body tissues, especially in the brain and nerve tissues, bile, blood, and the liver, where most of the cholesterol is synthesized.

The term **serum cholesterol** refers to the amount of cholesterol circulating in the blood. When serum cholesterol levels are high, cholesterol plaque builds up in the arteries and blocks blood circulation. This significantly increases the risk of heart disease.

Serum Cholesterol Levels

The federal government's National Cholesterol Education Program recommends that all adults 20 and older have their serum cholesterol levels checked with a simple blood test. Table 9-1 summarizes the recommendations. The numbers reported indicate milligrams of cholesterol per deciliter of blood (mg/dl).

Low- and High-Density Lipoproteins

Cholesterol is carried in the blood stream by fatty-cholesterol particles called lipoproteins. Two types of lipoproteins are involved in this process. These are:

- **low-density lipoprotein (LDL),** which is also known as bad cholesterol because it leads to plaque build-up.
- **high-density lipoprotein (HDL),** which is also known as good cholesterol because it helps to eliminate plaque build-up. Raising HDL *may* help protect against heart attack.
  A 1:3 LDL-to-HDL ratio is generally acceptable.

Levels under 200 are highly desirable. As blood cholesterol increases above this level, greater risk for heart disease occurs.

Levels between 200 and 239 indicate that dietary and lifestyle changes should be made. The levels should be rechecked by a physician within two months.

Levels above 240 indicate a risk for coronary heart disease and should be treated immediately.

TABLE 9-1   Serum Cholesterol Levels

Cholesterol management under medical supervision involves limiting dietary cholesterol, weight control, increasing exercise, and, if necessary, drug therapy.

Hypertension

Hypertension, which is commonly referred to as high blood pressure, is another major concern for adults because it is a major cause of heart attacks and strokes.

Blood Pressure Readings

Blood pressure is measured as two values: systolic pressure over diastolic pressure. **Systolic pressure,** which is the higher number, occurs when the ventricles of the heart contract and push the blood out from the heart. **Diastolic pressure,** which is the lower number, occurs when the ventricles of the heart relax.

Table 9-2 summarizes blood pressure recommendations. A patient with readings higher than these figures should be referred to his physician for evaluation.

In adults *under* 40 years of age, a reading of greater than 140/90 is considered to be hypertension.

In adults *over* 40 years of age, a reading of greater than 160/95 is considered to be hypertension.

TABLE 9-2 Blood Pressure Readings

Hypertension and Salt

When it comes to high blood pressure, salt is rapidly losing its reputation as "Public Enemy Number One." There is no evidence that excess salt can *cause* hypertension in healthy people. However, low-salt diets in combination with other measures are still recommended for all people *with* hypertension.

Many specialists now believe that other dietary factors such as insufficient calcium may set the stage for hypertension and may be even a more important factor than salt.

THE ELDERLY

The majority of the elderly, those persons 65 and older, are healthy and active; however, most also suffer from some of the chronic health problems associated with aging.

Factors Influencing Nutritional Status

Many reasons exist why some of the elderly have nutritional problems. These include:

- *Personal habits.* There appear to be many reasons why elderly individuals may impose upon themselves certain dietary restrictions. Unfortunately such restrictions can compromise nutritional status and ultimately place the individual at health risk.

- *Economic limitations.* Limited financial resources strongly influence food choices.
- *Sociological factors.* Living alone has a negative impact on food choices because of both the difficulty of getting out to shop and a decreased interest in fixing meals.
- *Physical limitations.* These limitations make it difficult to prepare meals. They may also limit a person's ability to chew and enjoy foods.
- *Medications.* The elderly are likely to be taking several medications on a long-term basis. These may influence the patient's nutritional needs.
- *Lack of knowledge.* Many of the elderly are not aware that good nutrition can still enhance their quality of life. Others lack knowledge of nutritional needs or do not know how to apply this information.
- *A "too late now" attitude.* Some elderly feel that it is too late to change to a more nutritious diet, but this is not true. Improved nutrition can be helpful throughout life.

The Effects of Lost Dentition

Declining chewing function may be an important reason why many of the elderly consume predominantly soft, easy-to-chew foods. This in turn can induce poor dietary practices and marginal nutrition intakes. Maintenance of chewing proficiency, through proper dental care, will help the individual enjoy a variety of foods that promote a state of nutritional well-being.

Special Nutritional Needs

The most recent RDA tables now include a category to reflect the needs of individuals over 51 years of age. In addition to these, the following nutritional guidelines are helpful when planning diets for this age group.

Energy Needs

Because of decreased activity, caloric needs usually decrease with age. Although energy needs are less, nutrient needs do not decrease. For this reason, it is particularly important to select foods with a high nutrient density and to avoid empty calories.

Protein

Protein needs do not change with age. Therefore, recommending either a high protein intake or a limited protein intake for the elderly is often inappropriate unless medical reasons necessitate it. Also excess dietary protein puts a strain on kidney function, which has decreased in many elderly.

Complex Carbohydrates

The consumption of complex carbohydrates, as well as fresh fruit, contributes to fiber intake. This is particularly important as intestinal activity decreases with age. In addition, complex carbohydrates contribute more vitamins and minerals than are found in most refined carbohydrates.

Refined Carbohydrates

Many older people tend to consume a higher proportion of refined carbohydrates in place of complex carbohydrates. This is because foods containing refined carbohydrates are readily available, simple to prepare, easy to eat, and lower in cost. These foods contain many empty calories and do not contribute significantly to the nutritional needs of the individual.

Fats

As with all ages, a decrease in fat is beneficial in reducing the possibility of obesity and cardiovascular disease.

Vitamins and Minerals

Because of dietary limitations and other factors, such as the interaction of medications, many of the elderly suffer vitamin and mineral deficiencies. If necessary, supplements may be recommended.

Osteoporosis

Osteoporosis is a condition in which there is an excessive loss of bone mass or density that results in weakening and brittleness of the bones. Eventually this weakening of the bones leads to fractures of the hip, wrist, ankle, and spine. Spinal fractures cause the disease's telltale rounded back and dowager's hump (Fig. 9-3).

This disorder afflicts older people, though women are more prone to it than men. In fact, it has been estimated that one-third of American women over 50 have osteoporosis.

Apparently, menopause marks the onset of an acute change in the calcium balance and rapid bone loss in women, with the most rapid bone loss occurring during the first five years following menopause.

Alveolar Bone Loss

Some researchers have suggested that the progressive loss of alveolar bone, leading to tooth loss, may be a manifes-

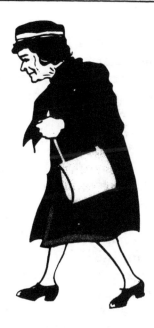

FIGURE 9-3 Osteoporosis may cause dowager's hump and a loss of height.

tation of osteoporosis. For example, they have found that women in their sixties with osteoporosis require new dentures because of excessive ridge resorption, three times as frequently as women who do not have osteoporosis.

Prevention

The prevention of osteoporosis begins early in life with the formation and maintenance of strong bones. Later in life a three-step prevention program is important.

1. *Exercise*, the kind which makes the muscles and bones work against gravity, can strengthen the skel-

eton. These are exercises such as walking, tennis, and running. Although swimming is an excellent aerobic exercise, it lacks the weight—bearing stress that builds bone mass.

2. *Adequate calcium intake* is essential throughout life. Before age 30 it helps to build bone mass. After age 30 it has a role in preventing calcium loss from the bones.

    The National Institute of Health recommends that women consume 1,000 milligrams of elemental calcium a day before menopause and 1,500 milligrams daily afterward. Women taking estrogen usually are advised to take 1,000 milligrams.

3. *Estrogen replacement therapy* slows the loss of calcium from the bones. It may also help protect postmenopausal women from heart attacks. However, the benefits of replacement hormones must be weighed against a possible increase in the patient's risk of certain cancers.

REVIEW EXERCISES _____

MULTIPLE CHOICE

Circle the correct answer for each question.

1. Formation of the permanent teeth usually begins by _____.

   a) the time the child is born
   b) three years of age
   c) early adolescence

2. Dipping the pacifier in honey may contribute to _____.

   a) baby bottle syndrome
   b) malformation of the jaw
   c) spoiling the baby

3. _____ nervosa is characterized by recurrent episodes of binge eating followed by purging to get rid of the food which was eaten.

   a) Anorexia
   b) Bulimia

4. Peak bone mass is probably achieved at about age _____.

   a) 15
   b) 25
   c) 35

5. A serum cholesterol level of under _____ is highly
    desirable.

    a) 200
    b) 250
    c) 300

6. Low-density lipoproteins are also known as _____
    cholesterol.

    a) bad
    b) good

7. In an adult under 40 years of age, a blood pressure
    reading of 140/90 is considered to be _____.

    a) borderline
    b) good news
    c) hypertension

8. Protein needs in most of the elderly _____ with
    age.

    a) decrease
    b) increase
    c) remain the same

9. Steps to prevent osteoporosis should begin _____.

    a) at menopause
    b) early in life
    c) when symptoms begin to appear

10. A patient with bulimia nervosa should be instructed to _____ after vomiting.

a) brush her teeth vigorously
b) rinse her mouth with an acid solution
c) rinse her mouth with an alkaline solution

SUGGESTED CLASS ACTIVITY

Discuss in class the special nutritional needs of different age groups and how they might be met. The discussion might include questions such as:

- What advice would you give a pregnant woman to help safeguard her health and the health of her baby?
- How would you explain BBS to a new parent?
- What steps can you take now to help prevent osteoporosis later?
- If you had to plan meals for your grandparents (or for imaginary grandparents), what sorts of problems could you expect to encounter in helping them meet their nutritional needs?

CHAPTER 10

SPECIAL DIETS FOR DENTAL PATIENTS

OBJECTIVES

After studying this chapter, you should be able to:

- describe a full liquid diet and list foods from each group that are included in this type of diet.
- describe a soft diet and list foods from each group that are included in this type of diet.
- differentiate between biting and chewing and explain why these differences are important in planning a diet for a dental patient.
- list the special dietary precautions that should be taken by a patient with a bonded veneer on an anterior tooth.
- describe the suggested dietary modifications for a patient with a fractured anterior tooth.

(Continued)

- list the types of foods that should be avoided by an orthodontic patient.
- describe the recommended dietary modifications for a patient with acute necrotizing gingivitis and one recovering from periodontal or oral surgery.
- describe the special dietary needs of a patient with wired jaws or severely limited mouth opening because of a temporomandibular joint disorder.
- describe the advice that might be given to a patient who is adjusting to a new denture.

INTRODUCTION TO SPECIAL DIETS

There are many reasons a dental patient might require a special or modified diet. However, before exploring the specifics it is important to understand the process that takes place in the body as a wound heals.

Wound Healing

The early stages of wound healing can take place effectively even in an extremely malnourished patient. The wound becomes the center of attention or "favored biological site." If necessary, the body may begin to draw from other body tissues to provide the necessary ingredients for early repair. At this stage the wound appears to have priority over almost all other metabolic processes.

After a suitable period, the length of which appears to be governed by time rather than degree of healing, the priority changes. The body begins to rebuild those tissues sacrificed for the wound repair. At this point the nutritional status and the level of current nutritional support become of primary importance to recovery.

The healing process is complex and requires the interaction of many critical biological processes. Because of this it is difficult to imagine a situation where some aspect of the healing process would not be impaired by an inadequate supply of any given nutrient.

It has not been proven conclusively that certain nutrients promote healing. It would be a more accurate concept to assume that any nutrient or nutrient combination that is not available in the correct concentration at the appropriate time may interfere with healing and recovery.

With an elective procedure (such as periodontal surgery) where there is a choice as to when the surgery will be performed, steps should be taken to ensure that the patient is well nourished prior to the procedure. After surgery, steps should be taken to be certain that the patient receives adequate nourishment despite impaired chewing ability.

TYPES OF SPECIAL DIETS

The goal of any special diet is to provide the patient with a well-balanced food intake that will meet nutritional needs in a form that can be comfortably consumed as well as appetizing.

The special diets that are most likely to be recommended for a dental patient who is not in a hospital setting are a full liquid diet, soft diet, or a modified diet.

Liquid Diets

A **clear liquid diet** consists of broths, gelatin, and clear liquids that the patient can consume comfortably. These foods are digested easily and leave no residue. This type of diet is most often used in a hospital setting and is not generally required by dental patients outside of that setting.

A **full liquid diet** is one that includes a wider range of foods. These are foods that are liquid at room temperature or that liquify at body temperature. A full liquid diet also includes foods that have been liquified by processing in a blender. A dental patient requiring a liquid diet is usually on it for only a few days. Table 10-1 is a list of the foods commonly included in a liquid diet.

Liquid formula foods are commercially available preparations that are prepared to include all necessary nutrients in a form that ranges from 300 to 3,000 calories per day. Depending on the patient's nutritional status, these foods may be prescribed for a period of time prior to and after surgery. They may also be used as dietary supplements. The type of formula food selected must take into consideration the patient's individual nutritional and energy needs.

Soft Diets

For dental patients, a soft diet is a modification of a normal diet. It eliminates foods that are difficult to chew. Table 10-2 lists the foods commonly included in a soft diet.

In discussing a soft diet, it is important to differentiate between biting and chewing.

- **Biting** requires the use of the anterior teeth to cut or tear food into bite-size pieces.
- **Chewing** requires the use of the posterior teeth to grind the food before it is swallowed.

Milk, yogurt, and cheese group	Milk (may be skim or low fat) Instant breakfast (mixed with milk) Plain yogurt (not with fruit) Eggnog Milk shake Cottage cheese (creamy style) Ice cream Pudding
Meat, poultry, fish, dried beans, eggs, and nuts group	Strained meat added to soup or broth Eggs, soft-cooked or scrambled Eggs in custard
Bread, cereal, rice, and pasta group	Cream of wheat cereal Cream of rice cereal Grits (thinned) Oatmeal (strained)
Vegetable group	Tomato juice Mixed vegetable juice Pureed vegetables Creamed soup, strained (such as cream of tomato)
Fruit group	All fruit juices Sherbets made with fruit juice Pureed fruits
Other	Flavored gelatin, plain (not with fruit) Carbonated beverages Coffee and tea Liquid dietary supplements

TABLE 10-1 Suggested Foods for a Liquid Diet

Milk, yogurt, and cheese group	All foods listed for a liquid diet Soft, mildly flavored cheeses Cream cheese
Meat, poultry, fish, dried beans, eggs, and nuts group	All foods listed for a liquid diet Very tender, ground, or pureed beef, veal, pork, ham, poultry, fish, or seafood Smooth peanut butter Soft meat casseroles Dried beans cooked very soft
Bread, cereal, rice, and pasta group	All foods listed for a liquid diet Soft breads (Avoid hard rolls, crisp toast, and bread with grains or seeds.) Pancakes, biscuits, hot bread Graham crackers Saltines (Avoid hard, crisp crackers.) Dry cereals softened in milk Soft cookies (Avoid nuts, raisins, and chocolate chips.)
Vegetable group	All foods listed for a liquid diet Cooked or canned vegetables (if tender and in small pieces) Mashed potatoes, white or sweet (Avoid fried potatoes and potato or corn chips.) Vegetable soup (with vegetables cooked very soft)
Fruit group	All foods listed for a liquid diet Applesauce Cooked or canned fruits (if soft and in small pieces) Ripe bananas Ripe fruit (if soft or mashed or cut into small pieces)
Other	All foods listed for a liquid diet

TABLE 10-2   Suggested Foods for a Soft Diet

Supplementation

For each patient requiring a special diet, the dentist will evaluate whether or not a diet supplement is desirable or necessary. The dentist may recommend dietary supplements depending upon:

- the patient's nutritional status prior to the surgery or injury.
- the length of time the patient will be on a restricted diet.
- the patient's ability to meet all nutritional requirements through diet during the recovery period.

MODIFIED DIETS

Bonded Veneers on Anterior Teeth

Patients who have had porcelain or composite veneers placed on their anterior teeth do not require a special diet; however, they should be cautioned against biting on foods that might fracture or damage this dental work.

Examples

- Avoid chewing on ice or other hard substances that may cause the veneer to fracture.
- Avoid biting into apples, carrots, or other very hard foods that could cause the veneer to fracture. These foods may be eaten, but they should be cut into bite-size pieces first.

Injured Anterior Teeth

Injured anterior teeth, such as those which have been badly bumped in an accident, must be protected from additional stress while they are healing. To accomplish this the patient is instructed to avoid biting hard foods. (Remember, biting involves use of the anterior teeth.)

Depending upon the severity of any accompanying lip or tongue injuries, the dentist may also recommend a liquid or soft diet for a few days. However, for most patients of this type the primary dietary modification is to avoid foods that require biting or tearing with the anterior teeth.

Examples

- Most foods that can be cut into small, bite-size pieces are acceptable.
- Fresh fruits can be included if they are cut into very small pieces that are chewed but not bitten.
- Since it is difficult to cut sandwiches into small enough pieces, it is best to avoid them. Soup and crackers (softened in the soup) are a good substitute.
- Hard toast, rolls, and pretzels (which require biting) should be avoided.

Wired Jaws

Patients with a fractured jaw or other problem that requires wiring the jaws together must get all of their nutrition through a full liquid diet. This is usually taken through a straw.

The patient should eat from five to six times a day and must be encouraged to drink an adequate amount of fluid (approximately two to three quarts daily) to keep from becoming dehydrated. This can be taken as water, juices, soft drinks, coffee, tea, and so on.

Because this diet is so limited, and because the jaws are usually wired for many weeks, it is advisable to have the patient's diet planned and managed under the supervision of a professional dietician.

Temporomandibular Joint Disorders

A patient with a temporomandibular joint disorder (TJD) may have pain when chewing and may be limited as to how wide the mouth can be opened. If jaw opening is severe, the patient may require a liquid diet. If the patient's mouth can be opened adequately but is painful when chewing, a soft diet may be indicated.

Orthodontic Patients

Nutritional Considerations in Orthodontics

Orthodontic tooth movement relies on the biological response of the periodontal ligament and alveolar bone to applied force systems. The literature suggests that the orthodontic patient's nutritional status can affect these biologic responses to orthodontic brackets and wires.

This tissue response is similar to healing in that it represents an additional challenge to the patient's body. Furthermore, the orthodontic patient is usually selectively treated during the adolescent growth spurt, which provides an additional challenge to the child's nutritional status.

Therefore, it is particularly important that the orthodontic patient be well nourished and in good health throughout treatment. At times when the teeth are sore (such as after banding or adjustments), the patient may want to eat a well-balanced soft diet until the discomfort has passed.

In addition, the orthodontic appliances themselves create special dietary problems. *First*, they trap food and shelter plaque. This makes oral hygiene particularly difficult and increases the importance of avoiding sticky cariogenic foods.

Second, orthodontic brackets, bands, wires, and appliances can be bent or damaged by very firm foods. Orthodontic patients should avoid anything that is sticky, gummy, chewy, or very hard (Fig. 10-1).

Examples of Foods to be Avoided

- Chewing gum
- Caramels, taffy, and all sticky candy
- Chewing on ice
- Jawbreakers or very hard candy
- Popcorn kernels (which may lodge under the braces and cause irritation)
- Biting into a raw apple or carrot (these may be eaten if cut into bite-size pieces)
- Biting on hard pretzels
- Corn on the cob
- Biting into hard bread or rolls

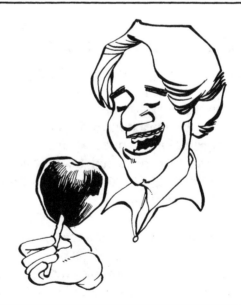

FIGURE 10-1 Orthodontic patients should avoid foods that are very sticky, highly cariogenic, or very hard.

Acute Necrotizing Ulcerative Gingivitis

A patient with acute necrotizing ulcerative gingivitis (ANUG) has a very sore mouth, does not feel well, and may not want to eat. However, good nutrition is essential to his recovery.

The following dietary modifications may be recommended to the ANUG patient:

- Eat a liquid or soft diet for the first few days.
- Avoid all spicy or irritating foods.
- Choose bland foods, such as gelatin and ice cream, that feel soothing.
- Eat frequent small meals.
- Drink plenty of fluids.
- Take dietary supplements as recommended by the dentist.

The Periodontal Surgery Patient

Following periodontal surgery, the patient has a two-part problem. *First,* his mouth is sore and biting is painful—yet maintaining good nutrition is essential to healing.

Second, the periodontal dressing which has been placed over the surgical area must be protected so that parts do not break off and food does not become lodged under it.

The following dietary modifications may be recommended to the patient:

- Avoid alcoholic beverages and foods that are spicy or irritating to the tissues.
- Drink only cold liquids during the first 24 hours. This will help the dressing to harden properly and will also help to prevent swelling.
- Eat a soft diet for the first 24 to 48 hours until some of the soreness begins to go away. After that, and

until the dressing is removed, avoid hard foods that require a lot of chewing.
- Avoid popcorn or anything with husks that may get under the dressing.
- Avoid very hard and crunchy foods, such as large pieces of raw fruits or vegetables, that may cause the dressing to break.
- Avoid sticky foods that might stick to the dressing.

The Oral Surgery Patient

The special problems faced by a patient after oral surgery are the possibility of reduced appetite, a desire to protect the wound site, and the inability to chew in the area of the surgery. Depending upon the extent of the surgery, the patient may require a liquid or soft diet for the first few days.

The following are general recommendations for oral surgery patients. (In extensive cases, the dentist may make more specific recommendations.)

- During the first several days, take special care not to disturb the blood clot and surgical area when you eat or drink.
- Drink plenty of liquids.
- Eat soft foods during the first 12 to 24 hours.
- After this period, eat as normally as possible by chewing on the other side.
- Avoid alcoholic beverages, spicy foods, and hot liquids that may be irritating.

The New Denture Patient

The transition from natural to artificial teeth requires a period of adjustment as the patient learns to speak, bite, and chew with the new denture.

Although a special diet is not required, the following are some dietary suggestions that can be made to the patient to aid in this adjustment:

- Cut regular food into small pieces.
- Take small bites and chew slowly.
- At first, avoid sticky or very hard foods.
- Chew foods on both sides with the back teeth. This will prevent tipping of the denture.
- Be careful. With the denture in place your mouth will be less sensitive to very hot temperatures. Until you have adjusted to this, take special care to avoid very hot foods and liquids that could burn your mouth.

The Immediate Denture Patient

The patient with an immediate denture has a two-part problem. *First,* he is recovering from surgery (the extraction of the remaining teeth). *Second,* he must adjust to the new denture. This patient may require a soft or liquid diet for the first few days. After this, he should be encouraged to follow the suggestions for other new denture patients.

REVIEW EXERCISES _____

MULTIPLE CHOICE

Circle the correct answer for each question.

1. _____ is suggested for a liquid diet.

   a) Applesauce
   b) Dried cereal softened in milk
   c) Plain yogurt

2. A patient with injured anterior teeth should avoid eating a sandwich because it requires _____.

   a) biting
   b) chewing
   c) a and b

3. Orthodontic patients should avoid eating _____.

   a) all raw fruits
   b) all raw vegetables
   c) corn on the cob

4. A patient with wired jaws should _____.

   a) avoid hot and spicy foods
   b) have his diet planned by a professional dietician
   c) use a commercially available liquid diet product

5. A patient with a bonded anterior veneer should _____.

   a) avoid foods that might fracture the veneer
   b) avoid very hot or spicy foods
   c) eat only a soft diet

6. During the early stages of wound healing, the body gives the wound _____.

   a) favored biological status
   b) priority over almost all other metabolic processes
   c) a and b

7. A patient with _____ should select bland foods such as gelatin and ice cream.

   a) a temporomandibular disorder
   b) ANUG
   c) wired jaws

8. Following periodontal surgery, the patient should drink only _____ liquids during the first 24 hours.

   a) cold
   b) hot

9. Fried potatoes _____ included in a soft diet.

   a) are
   b) are not

10. A new denture wearer should _____.

    a) avoid sandwiches
    b) cut food into small pieces
    c) eat a soft diet for the first few days

SUGGESTED CLASS ACTIVITY

Pretend that you were in an accident and injured your anterior teeth. (Fortunately you have no cut lip or other serious injuries.) Plan a diet for yourself for three days that will fill your nutritional needs without further injuring these teeth.

CHAPTER 11

THE ROLE OF FLUORIDES IN PREVENTIVE DENTISTRY

OBJECTIVES _____

After studying this chapter, you should be able to:

- differentiate between systemic and topical fluorides.
- discuss the safety of fluorides and identify one major area of concern.
- describe the role of fluorides during tooth development.
- describe the process of remineralization.

(Continued)

- list at least four types of patients at high risk for dental decay.
- state the safe fluoride-to-water ratio.
- state at least three situations in which the dentist might prescribe dietary fluoride supplements.
- describe the use of topical fluoride gels both in the dental office and at home.
- discuss the use of fluoride mouth rinses.
- discuss the use of fluoride-containing toothpastes and state the special precautions that should be taken when children use these products.

OVERVIEW OF FLUORIDES

Fluorides, which are a nutrient, have been proven to be a very effective and safe means of preventing dental decay. The dramatic reduction of dental decay since the introduction of fluorides is one of the greatest public health success stories of this century.

Maximum benefits are achieved when both systemic and topical fluorides are available to work together.

Systemic and Topical Fluorides

Systemic fluorides, which are also known as **dietary fluorides**, are those ingested in water, food, beverages, or supplements. The required amount of fluoride is absorbed through the intestine into the bloodstream. Any excess is excreted by the body through the skin, kidneys, and feces.

Topical fluorides, which are also known as **non-dietary fluorides**, are those which are applied directly to the teeth through mouth rinses, fluoridated toothpastes, and topical fluoride applications.

The Safety of Fluorides

Fluoride in excessive amounts is poisonous. However, the levels of fluoride in controlled water fluoridation are so low that there is little danger of ingesting an acutely toxic quantity of fluoride from fluoridated water.

In some areas fluoride occurs naturally in the water in extremely high amounts. This may cause **dental fluorosis,** which is also known as **mottled enamel.** Mild fluorosis may appear as white spots on the teeth. In severe cases, the enamel is discolored and badly weakened.

In contrast to the safety of fluoridated water, an area of concern is having young children ingest excessive fluorides by eating fluoridated toothpaste or swallowing fluoride rinses or topical gels. Patients should use fluoride preparations only as recommended by the dentist and should supervise their use by young children.

How Fluorides Help Teeth

Prenatal Development

In large part, the strength and structure of the teeth depends on the nutrients available to the developing child. All of these nutrients must come from the mother's diet. If the mother is ingesting dietary fluorides, some of these are also used by the baby.

Birth to Three Years

During the period between birth and three years of age, all the crowns of the primary teeth and most of the crowns of the permanent teeth have either finished mineralizing or are in the process of completing their mineralization.

Throughout this period, systemic fluoride is incorporated into the developing teeth and helps to make them more caries resistant. Newly-erupted teeth are incompletely mineralized and further uptake of minerals and fluoride from saliva and food occurs shortly after eruption. This further increases the caries resistance of the teeth.

Fluorides Throughout Life

When fluorides were first introduced, it was thought they were helpful only during the developmental period of the teeth. However, research has now shown that it is also essential to have an ongoing source of fluoride throughout life.

In the past it was believed that if minerals were lost from a tooth through a process called **demineralization**, the lesion could not be repaired. However, research has shown that if an ongoing source of fluoride is available, **remineralization** may occur (Table 11-1).

Remineralization is able to reverse the damage of early demineralization. However, if the lesion has progressed too far, remineralization cannot halt the process, and it is necessary to repair the tooth with a dental restoration.

High-Risk Patients

For most patients, the combination of fluoridated water and fluoridated toothpaste is very effective in preventing dental decay. However, high-risk patients who are particularly prone to dental decay may require additional sources

Demineralization	Acid from dental plaque causes minerals (particularly calcium and phosphate) to be lost from enamel.
White spot lesion	The demineralized area is white in appearance and is known as a white spot lesion. This is the first step toward decay.
Remineralization	Fluoride in the saliva works with calcium and phosphate (also found in saliva) to encourage the formation of new crystals to remineralize the damaged area.

TABLE 11-1

such as topical applications and fluoride rinses. The category of high-risk patients is summarized in Table 11-2.

SYSTEMIC FLUORIDES

Fluoridated Water

Fluoride added to public water supplies is an effective, practical, and cost-effective caries-reducing measure. According to 1991 figures released by the U.S. Public Health Service, over a 75-year life span the per individual cost of adding fluoride to the public drinking water was far less than the cost of a single dental restoration.

The safe fluoride-to-water ratio is one **part per million (ppm)**. This means one part of fluoride to one million parts of water. It is approximately the equivalent of one drop of fluoride in a bathtub full of water. This optimal amount varies

Some, but not all, patients living in areas where the public water supply is not fluoridated.

Patients with a history of dental decay.

Adults who are prone to root caries. (Root caries are decay that occurs on the root of the tooth that has been exposed because of the loss of gingival tissue due to periodontal disease.)

Patients with illnesses, or taking medications, which slow the flow of saliva.

Patients undergoing chemotherapy or radiation treatment which damages the tissues and affects the flow of saliva.

Patients who are anorexic or bulimic.

Patients who have had periodontal surgery which leaves the root surface exposed and sensitive.

TABLE 11-2   High-Risk Dental Patients

(from 0.7 to 1.2 ppm) depending on the climate and average temperature of the community.

In-Home Water Filters

In communities with a fluoridated water supply, some in-home water filters may remove the fluoride. When this happens, the family will not receive the benefits of the fluoridated water. Fluoride is removed from water through reverse osmosis, distillation, and carbonated alumina home water treatment systems. Fluoride is not removed from the water with ion exchange/softeners, sediment filters, and ultraviolet systems.

Bottled Water

Unless the fluoride content is printed on the label, it is not safe to assume that bottled water contains adequate fluoride to prevent dental decay. If only bottled water without fluoride is used for drinking and cooking, the family may not receive the full benefits of systemic fluoride.

Prescribed Dietary Fluoride Supplements

Dietary fluoride supplements, in the form of drops or tablets, may be prescribed by the dentist. The following are some of the situations in which the dentist may consider prescribing a supplement.

Drinking Water Below Optimal Level of Fluoride

A primary use of prescribed dietary fluoride supplements is for patients living in areas where the drinking water is below the optimal level of fluoride. However, before prescribing a supplement, the dentist must determine the fluoride level of the family drinking water supply.

Information about the fluoride content of the public water supply can be obtained by contacting the local water department. If the water source is a private well, a water sample can be sent to the local or county health department for a fluoride content analysis.

Prenatal Fluorides

If the mother is living in an area where fluoridated water is not available, the dentist may recommend that the mother take fluoride supplements as a means of helping the baby develop stronger teeth.

Breast Milk and Formula

Fluoride consumed by the mother does not pass into breast milk. Since breast milk does not contain fluoride, a baby who is only breast-fed may not receive enough fluoride. If a baby is fed only ready-to-use formula that does not contain fluoride, or if the formula is mixed with water that does not contain fluoride, the baby may not receive sufficient dietary fluoride. In these situations the dentist may prescribe a fluoride supplement for the child.

Starting Early

The effectiveness of these supplements is greater the earlier the child begins to take them. However, their effectiveness also depends on daily administration over a long period of time. This requires a very high level of parental motivation.

Dietary supplements of fluoride may be the method of choice for the very young child. For older children, topical fluoride application or fluoride mouth rinses often may be preferable. Children who are highly susceptible to caries may benefit from receiving both measures.

Cautions

As with all medicines, there is a danger if a child ingests a large quantity. Therefore, as a precautionary measure the dentist will prescribe only a limited amount of fluoride to be dispensed at one time. Each package of fluoride supplement should be labeled: *Caution—store out of reach of children.*

TOPICAL FLUORIDES

Professional Application of Topical Fluorides

Professional topical fluoride applications have been proven effective for some children soon after the eruption of the permanent teeth. These applications are also recommended for some high-risk patients. The frequency of professional topical applications depends on the patient's needs and on the type of fluoride used.

The most commonly used topical fluoride is an acidulated fluoride gel that is easily applied in a disposable tray after the patient's teeth have been thoroughly cleaned. (A dental auxiliary may be assigned this task.)

Because of the danger of ingesting excessive fluoride, the patient must be cautioned not to swallow the fluoride solution. However, to maximize the benefit of the fluoride the patient is advised not to rinse for 30 minutes after the treatment.

Brush-on Fluoride Gel

A 1.1 percent neutral sodium fluoride brush-on gel is available without prescription. A two percent neutral sodium fluoride brush-on gel is available by prescription. High-risk patients may use these at home by brushing them or through home application with a reusable custom tray.

The custom tray for applying these gels is made in the dental office using a vacuum former working with a diagnostic cast of the patient's mouth. In order to bring the fluoride gel into close contact with all of the tooth surfaces the tray is designed to cover the teeth and to extend slightly beyond the gingival margin.

The patient is instructed to use the tray at bedtime. A

small amount of the brush-on gel is placed in the tray and the tray is placed over the teeth for five minutes. If water in the area is fluoridated, the patient is instructed to rinse and spit. This prevents ingestion of excess fluoride. If water in the area is not fluoridated, the patient is told not to rinse after the application. Any fluoride that is swallowed will provide extra dietary fluoride.

Fluoride Mouth Rinses

Mouth rinses containing fluoride are another way of providing fluorides to those in areas without fluoridated water and for patients with special needs. Over-the-counter non-prescriptive rinses generally contain .05 percent sodium fluoride (NaF). They are designed to be used on a daily basis. Prescription rinses generally contain .2 percent sodium fluoride. They are designed to be used once a week.

Because of the danger of ingesting excessive fluoride, the patient must be cautioned not to swallow the mouth rinse. Fluoride mouth rinses are *not* usually recommended for children under five years of age or for some handicapped children because they may swallow the rinse rather than spit it out.

Fluoride-Containing Toothpastes

Toothpastes containing fluoride are an important ongoing source of topical fluorides; today most dentifrices contain fluoride. A major benefit of these fluorides is the brushing action that brings them into close contact with all surfaces of the teeth.

Cautions

However, because of the danger of ingesting excessive fluoride, the patient should be cautioned not to swallow or eat the toothpaste. Caution is particularly important for very young children (under four years of age) who have difficulty rinsing their mouths and spitting out the excess. For these children, particularly those who are receiving fluorides from other sources, the dentist may recommend the following steps:

- Use a child-size toothbrush.
- Use a pea-sized amount of toothpaste on the toothbrush.
- Brush under the supervision of a parent or other responsible person.
- Do not swallow the toothpaste.

REVIEW EXERCISES _____

MULTIPLE CHOICE
Circle the correct answer for each question.

1. Fluoride is a _____.

    a) nutrient
    b) poison
    c) a and b

2. Remineralization is able to reverse _____.

    a) demineralization
    b) fluorosis
    c) mottled enamel

3. The safe fluoride-to-water ratio for fluoridated water is _____ part(s) per million.

    a) one
    b) ten
    c) one hundred

4. To increase their dietary fluoride intake, children should be encouraged to swallow fluoridated rinses.

    a) true
    b) false

5. Bottled water contains _____ fluoride.

    a) adequate
    b) no
    c) a label which may indicate the amount of

6. After a professional topical fluoride application in the dental office, the patient is advised to _____.

a) rinse his mouth immediately.
b) swallow the fluoride
c) wait 30 minutes before rinsing his mouth

7. If the mother drinks fluoridated water, breast milk _____ contain fluoride.

a) does
b) does not

8. A major benefit of fluorides in toothpaste is _____.

a) brushing brings the fluoride into close contact with the teeth
b) they serve as a source of dietary fluoride
c) a and b

9. If the community water supply is not fluoridated, the dentist will prescribe dietary supplements _____.

a) after determining the fluoride level of the family's drinking water supply
b) for all patients
c) routinely for school age children

10. A patient who has an illness or is taking medication that slows the flow of saliva _____ at high risk for dental decay.

a) is
b) is not

SUGGESTED CLASS ACTIVITY

Talk with your parents, grandparents, or another older individual who grew up before fluorides were used as a preventive dentistry measure. Ask what it was like to grow up in a time when most children routinely had many cavities. (Do you imagine these children were happy dental patients?)

How has this early decay affected each individual's dental health today? How different do you think their dental health would be now if they had had the benefits of fluorides throughout their lives?

CHAPTER 12

THE ROLE OF PLAQUE CONTROL IN PREVENTIVE DENTISTRY

OBJECTIVES _____

After studying this chapter, you should be able to:

- describe dental plaque and discuss its role in dental disease.
- discuss the role of cariogenic foods in relation to dental plaque.
- differentiate between cariogenic, noncariogenic, and anti-cariogenic foods. Also give an example of each type of food.
- demonstrate the use of disclosing tablets or solution.

(Continued)

> • discuss the criteria for toothbrush selection.
> • demonstrate the toothbrushing and flossing techniques as recommended by the American Academy of Periodontology.

DENTAL PLAQUE

Dental plaque, is a sticky, soft deposit consisting chiefly of bacteria and bacterial products. It also contains food debris and components from the saliva. The bacteria in plaque convert sugars from carbohydrates into acid. This acid attacks the enamel of the tooth and may cause demineralization as described in Chapter 11.

Small amounts of plaque cannot be seen easily. However, as plaque accumulates, it becomes visible and ranges in color from gray to yellowish-gray to yellow.

Most frequently plaque buildup occurs in sheltered areas where the natural cleansing mechanisms of the mouth, such as the flow of saliva, the chewing of food, and the movement of the tongue do not disturb it. These areas are primarily around the necks of the teeth, between the teeth, and on the lingual (inner) surfaces of the upper posterior teeth. Plaque also accumulates on dental restorations and fixed bridges, as well as full and partial removable dentures.

The Types of Bacteria in Plaque

The types of bacteria contained in the plaque change constantly throughout the period of plaque development.

- **Facultative organisms**, bacteria that can thrive in either the presence or the absence of oxygen, are found most often in the early stages of plaque development.
- **Anaerobic organisms**, bacteria that thrive in the absence of oxygen, are found most often in more mature plaque.

Because of the differences in the types of bacteria in the plaque, it is possible to look at the plaque under a microscope and determine which are newly-formed colonies and which have been in place longer. This information is helpful in demonstrating to the patient which areas he is missing consistently in his plaque removal efforts.

Calculus

If not removed regularly, plaque deposits bond with minerals in saliva to form **calculus**, also known as **tartar**. These hardened deposits build up on the teeth and under the gum line and can only be removed through a dental prophylaxis. A **dental prophylaxis** is the professional cleaning of the teeth by the dentist or hygienist to remove plaque, calculus, and stains.

Plaque Removal

Fresh plaque, which has not calcified, can be removed by the patient through toothbrushing and flossing. Research has shown that once plaque has been removed, it takes approximately 24 hours to form and organize again. Therefore, it is important that all plaque be removed at least once every day. The means of removing plaque are discussed later in this chapter.

FOOD AND DENTAL PLAQUE

Foods contribute to plaque formation and acid attacks on the teeth in two ways. The *first* is through the types of foods eaten. The bacteria can only utilize certain types of foods. These foods are said to be cariogenic. The *second* factor is the frequency of eating cariogenic foods. Each time a cariogenic food is eaten it is converted into acid that attacks the teeth. Each episode is referred to as an **acid attack**.

Foods utilized by plaque are said to be **cariogenic**, which means causing decay. However, cariogenic is a relative term; it actually encompasses three types of food. These are:

- **anti-cariogenic** or **cariostatic** foods, which have been found to inhibit decay.
- **noncariogenic** foods, which do not promote tooth decay.
- **cariogenic** foods, which are most likely to cause decay.

Anti-Cariogenic Foods

Some foods are believed to have properties which inhibit the acid attack on the teeth. These foods include:

- certain types of cheese such as aged cheddar, Monterey Jack, and Swiss cheese.
- licorice.
- chocolate and other cocoa products.

Although these foods may not be harmful to the dentition, their intake must be considered in terms of their total nutritional value. For example, chocolate has a high caloric content from fat and sugar without providing other essential nutrients.

Noncariogenic Foods

Neither proteins nor fats provide an energy source for oral bacteria. If eaten by themselves these foods are non-cariogenic. However, most foods are eaten with, or processed to contain, either cooked starches or sugars that are cariogenic. In these combinations they, too, have the potential to contribute to acid formation.

A hot dog eaten on a roll with ketchup is an example of such a combination. The roll is a refined carbohydrate, and the ketchup contains sugar. The hot dog itself is a source of protein, a lot of fat, and may contain a cereal filler.

Cariogenic Foods

Carbohydrates are the only nutrients that are cariogenic because they are broken down in the mouth into sugars that the bacteria are able to utilize. The bacteria in plaque require only a small amount of sugar to start producing acid. Therefore the amount of sugars in a food is not the only factor related to its ability to cause acid formation.

To plaque bacteria, all sugars are essentially the same. **Simple carbohydrates** such as refined sugars, the sweeteners added to processed foods, and the sugars occurring naturally in honey and fruit are readily available to the bacteria.

Fermentable carbohydrates are complex carbohydrates, such as starch, that stay in the mouth long enough to be broken down into sugars by the action of the salivary amylase. (This is discussed in Chapter 2.)

Examples of fermentable carbohydrates are soft crackers, breakfast cereals, potato chips, dried fruit, and bread. Although these foods are not very sweet, they may stick to the teeth and remain in the mouth long enough to begin to be converted into sugars.

The Frequency of Eating

It appears to be the *frequency* of eating cariogenic foods and their *retentiveness* that are the major dietary factors in the decay process. Each time a cariogenic food is eaten, it is followed by an acid attack. The frequency of eating, particularly snacking, obviously increases the frequency of these attacks (Fig. 12-1).

Snacks that are often overlooked in terms of their impact on dental health include:

- coffee sweetened with sugar or with coffee lightener. (Most lighteners contain sugar.)
- chewing gum sweetened with sugar. Chewing sugar-free gum does not cause this problem.

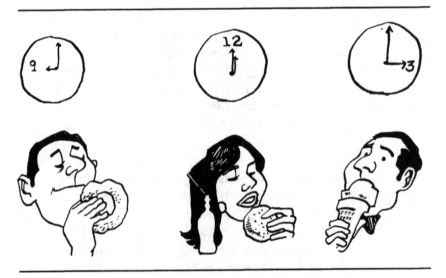

FIGURE 12-1 An acid attack occurs every time a cariogenic food is eaten. Each attack lasts at least 20 minutes.

- snack foods, such as pretzels, that may stick to the teeth long enough to be converted into sugars that can be used by the bacteria in plaque.
- hard candies, lifesavers, or breath mints that take a long time to consume and to clear the mouth.

Retentiveness

Retentiveness, which is also known as oral clearance time, refers to how long it takes the food to leave the mouth. A major factor here is the "stickiness" of the carbohydrate. Liquids have the most rapid clearance time and are least harmful, even though they may contain high percentages of sucrose.

A food's ability to stimulate salivary flow increases its speed of oral clearance. Some foods, such as caramel candy, which are thought of as being sticky, actually clear the mouth fairly quickly because they stimulate the flow of saliva. However, foods which combine starches and sugars often take longer to chew and may be retained around the teeth so that they are slow to clear the mouth. For this reason they are generally more cariogenic than foods which contain sugars alone.

PERSONAL ORAL HYGIENE (POH)

The phrase "personal oral hygiene" encompasses all of the techniques used by the patient at home to remove and control dental plaque. The patient learns these techniques in the dental office. When working with a patient in this type of teaching situation, it is necessary to establish a setting that is comfortable and supportive. In this setting the "teacher" should be accepting, not critical, and work to help the patient acquire the necessary skills.

An important goal of this instruction is to involve the patient fully so that any problems will be recognized and solved. It is also very important that the teacher be a good role model by following a home-care program that maintains good oral hygiene and by receiving regular professional care as necessary.

A personal oral hygiene program usually includes:

- the use of disclosing agents to help the patient understand the plaque problem.
- learning the toothbrushing technique recommended by the dentist. Brushing helps to remove retained food and is an important first step in plaque removal.
- learning the flossing technique recommended by the dentist. Flossing removes plaque from the sheltered places around the necks of the teeth and between the teeth.
- learning to use other home-care aids as recommended by the dentist.

Disclosing Agents

Since plaque is hard to see, it must be made visible so that the patient can see what needs to be removed. A **red disclosing tablet** is used for this purpose. This tablet consists of a harmless dye that will rinse off the tongue, teeth, and lips. Swallowing the solution will not harm the patient; however, it is recommended that the patient spit out the excess solution. The patient should chew one tablet and swish the liquid around in the mouth for at least 30 seconds. Then the mouth should be rinsed twice with plain water. The red-colored areas remaining on the teeth indicate plaque, which must be removed.

Disclosing tablets are used daily during the first week. After this, they are used periodically as needed to check the effectiveness of the plaque removal efforts.

Toothbrush Selection

The toothbrush selected should:

- have soft, round-ended bristles.
- be small enough to fit comfortably into the patient's mouth.
- have a handle that enables the patient to move it about easily.

Toothbrushes wear out. The bristles may become bent and the ends fray. When this happens, the toothbrush can no longer clean effectively and should be replaced.

Toothpastes

Toothpastes, also known as **dentifrices**, are aids for cleaning and polishing tooth surfaces.

Toothpastes with Fluorides

Those toothpastes containing fluorides (sodium mono-fluorophosphate, sodium fluoride, or stannous fluoride) provide added protection to the teeth. This is discussed in Chapter 11.

To be most effective in providing fluorides, these toothpastes must come into close contact with the teeth. This goal is best achieved by placing the paste *between* the bristles of the toothbrush. If the paste is placed only on top of the bristles, most of it is rinsed away before it reaches the tooth surfaces.

Tartar Control Toothpastes

Some toothpastes contain chemicals that slow the buildup of tartar. Although they may help prevent a buildup, they cannot remove any tartar that is already present. If all plaque is removed daily, there will not be a tartar buildup.

Toothpastes to Whiten Teeth

Some toothpastes advertise their special ability to whiten teeth. The patient may want to ask the dentist about using these pastes since they may be more abrasive than other toothpastes. Those containing peroxide bleach may be irritating to the oral tissues if used over a long period of time.

Toothbrushing Technique

When a patient is learning a new toothbrushing technique, he should practice first without putting toothpaste on the brush. The reason for this is because toothpaste foams, making it difficult to see what is happening during brushing. It is also helpful if he watches in the mirror to be certain that all surfaces of each tooth have been brushed thoroughly.

Once the new technique has been mastered, the patient will once again want to use fluoride-containing toothpaste. However, all patients should be cautioned against eating or swallowing excess fluoride containing toothpaste.

There are many methods of toothbrushing. The one described below is the technique recommended by the American Academy of Periodontology in their publication *How To Brush and Floss* (Chicago, 1989).

To Clean the Outer Surface of the Teeth

1. Position the brush horizontally at a 45-degree angle where the gums and teeth meet (Fig. 12-2).
2. Gently move the brush back and forth several times using small, circular strokes.

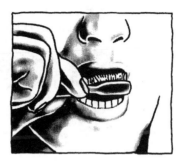

FIGURE 12-2   To brush the outside surface of the teeth, position the brush at a 45-degree angle.

3. Apply light pressure to get the bristles between the teeth, but do not use enough pressure to cause discomfort.
4. Change the position of the brush and repeat this motion as often as necessary to reach and clean all of the outer surfaces of the teeth.

To Clean the Inner Surface of the Back Teeth

1. For the back teeth, position the brush horizontally at a 45-degree angle where the gums and teeth meet (Fig. 12-3).
2. Gently move the brush back and forth several times using small, circular strokes.
3. Change the position of the brush and repeat this motion as often as necessary to reach and clean all of the inner surfaces of the upper and lower posterior teeth.

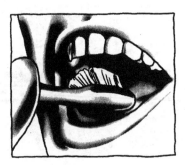

FIGURE 12-3 To brush the inside surface of the back
teeth, position the brush at a 45-degree angle.

To Clean the Inner Surface of the Front Teeth

1. To clean the inner surfaces of the upper and lower
    front teeth, hold the brush vertically (Fig. 12-4).
2. Make several gentle back-and-forth strokes over
    each tooth and its surrounding gum tissue.
3. Change the position of the brush and repeat this
    motion as often as necessary to reach and clean
    all of the inner surfaces of the upper and lower
    front teeth.
4. Closing the lips lightly around the toothbrush will
    help to prevent splashing.

To Clean the Chewing Surface of the Teeth

1. Place the bristles of the brush on the chewing
    surface and move the brush using small, circular
    strokes (Fig. 12-5).
2. Change the position of the brush and repeat this
    motion as often as necessary to reach and clean
    all of the chewing surfaces of the upper and lower
    teeth.

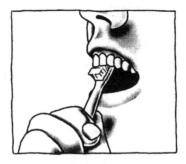

FIGURE 12-4 To clean the inner surface of the upper and lower front teeth, hold the brush vertically.

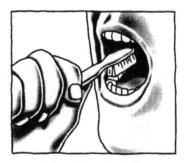

FIGURE 12-5 To clean the chewing surface of the teeth, use small, circular strokes.

To Rinse

1. After brushing, rinse vigorously to remove loosened plaque and debris.

Flossing

Dental floss is an effective way to remove plaque from spaces and surfaces *between* the teeth. The following are flossing instructions suggested by the American Academy of Periodontology in their publication *How To Brush and Floss* (Chicago, 1989).

Preparation

1. Cut a piece of waxed or unwaxed floss about 18 inches long.
2. Wrap most of the floss lightly around the middle finger of one hand. Wrap the rest of the floss lightly around the middle finger of the opposite hand (Fig. 12-6).

Flossing the Upper Teeth

1. Hold the floss tightly between the thumb and forefinger of each hand.
2. The fingers controlling the floss should be no more than one-half inch apart.
3. Gently pass the floss between the teeth using a sawing motion. Do not force or snap it into place (Fig. 12-7).
4. Guide the floss to the gumline. Curve the floss into a C-shape against one tooth. Gently slide it into the space between the gum and the tooth (Fig. 12-8).
5. Using both hands, move the floss up and down on the side of one tooth.
6. Repeat this technique on each side of all the upper teeth including the back surface of the last tooth in each quadrant.
7. As the floss becomes frayed or soiled, move a fresh area into the working position.

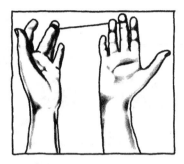

FIGURE 12-6 Loosely wrap the floss around the middle finger of each hand as shown.

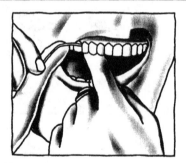

FIGURE 12-7 Gently pass the floss between the teeth using a sawing motion.

Flossing the Lower Teeth

1. Guide the floss using the forefingers of both hands (Fig. 12-9).
2. Gently pass the floss between the teeth using a sawing motion. Do not force or snap it into place.

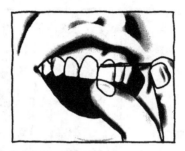

FIGURE 12-8 Curve the floss into a C-shape
against the tooth.

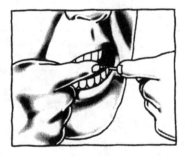

FIGURE 12-9 When flossing the lower teeth, use the
forefingers of both hands to guide the floss.

3. Guide the floss to the gumline. Curve the floss into a
   C-shape against one tooth. Gently slide it into the
   space between the gum and the tooth.
4. Using both hands, move the floss up and down on
   the side of one tooth.
5. Repeat this technique on each side of all the lower
   teeth including the back surface of the last tooth in
   each quadrant (Fig. 12-10).

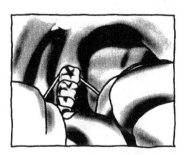

FIGURE 12-10 Wrap the floss into a C-shape around the back of the last tooth in each quadrant.

6. As the floss becomes frayed or soiled, move a fresh area into the working position.

Rinsing Again

1. Rinse vigorously after flossing. Recheck with disclosing solution.

Other Aids

Interproximal Brushes

Interproximal brushes are very small brushes, usually triangular in shape, that can be attached to a handle. These are recommended for cleaning between teeth with large or open interdental spaces. These spaces may occur if there is gingival recession or if the patient has required periodontal treatment. The brush is slipped between the teeth near the gum line. Here it is moved back-and-forth in short strokes.

Stim-U-Dents

A Stim-U-Dent is a brand name for a soft wooden tip that is triangular in cross section. It is moistened prior to use and is held between the middle finger, index finger, and thumb. The Stim-U-Dent is gently introduced between the teeth near the gingival surface and the tip is gently forced in and out of the space to provide a cleaning and massaging action.

Antimicrobial Rinses

The dentist may prescribe an antimicrobial oral rinse for some patients with periodontal problems. This rinse, which is used twice daily, contains chlorhexidine gluconate 0.12 percent.

The purpose of the rinse is to reduce the concentration of some bacteria in the saliva. Because the solution may affect the taste of certain foods, it is generally recommended that it be used after meals. These rinses also stain the teeth; however, these stains can be removed with professional cleaning.

Mouthwashes

Most people use nonprescription mouthwashes to freshen their breath; however, these substances mask the problem only briefly and do not cure it. "Bad breath" may be caused by many factors including:

- periodontal disease, especially when accompanied by bleeding gums.
- respiratory-tract infections such as chronic bronchitis or sinusitis with postnasal drip.
- aromatic compounds in foods like garlic and onions. These enter the bloodstream and are carried to the lungs, then exhaled.
- decreased saliva flow during sleep.

REVIEW EXERCISES _____

MULTIPLE CHOICE

Circle the correct answer for each question.

1. A _____ food does not promote dental decay.

   a) cariogenic
   b) fermentable carbohydrate
   c) noncariogenic

2. When the patient is learning a new toothbrushing technique, he should be encouraged to brush _____ toothpaste.

   a) with
   b) without

3. A/An _____ organism thrives in the absence of oxygen.

   a) anaerobic
   b) facultative

4. Calculus can be removed _____.

   a) daily with careful toothbrushing
   b) only by a professional dental prophylaxis
   c) through the use of an antitartar toothpaste

5. All dental plaque should be removed _____.

   a) after every meal
   b) at least once every 24 hours
   c) by the dental hygienist

6. Chocolate is a/an _____ food.

   a) anti-cariogenic
   b) cariogenic
   c) noncariogenic

7. A _____ carbohydrate is one that stays in the mouth long enough to be acted upon by the salivary amylase.

   a) fermentable
   b) simple

8. The bacteria in plaque _____ able to utilize fats and protein as food.

   a) are
   b) are not

9. A disclosing agent is used to _____.

   a) make plaque visible
   b) speed oral clearance
   c) stop an acid attack

10. When cleaning the inner surfaces of the front teeth, the toothbrush is held _____.

    a) at a 45 degree angle
    b) horizontally
    c) vertically

SUGGESTED CLASS ACTIVITY

Be sure you have the following materials for personal oral hygiene: toothbrush, toothpaste, disclosing tablets, and dental floss. Work in pairs taking turns demonstrating how you perform the personal oral hygiene steps.

Now take turns *instructing* your partner in how to perform the personal oral hygiene steps.

After this, discuss how it felt to give a demonstration, to watch a demonstration, to teach these techniques, and to be taught these techniques.

APPENDIX   A

ANSWER KEYS _____

Chapter 1

1.	b)	6.	a)
2.	a)	7.	b)
3.	b)	8.	c)
4.	b)	9.	b)
5.	a)	10.	c)

Chapter 4

1.	c)	6.	b)
2.	a)	7.	b)
3.	b)	8.	c)
4.	b)	9.	a)
5.	b)	10.	a)

Chapter 2

1.	a)	6.	c)
2.	b)	7.	b)
3.	c)	8.	a)
4.	c)	9.	b)
5.	b)	10.	b)

Chapter 5

1.	a)	6.	b)
2.	c)	7.	a)
3.	b)	8.	a)
4.	c)	9.	c)
5.	c)	10.	a)

Chapter 3

1.	a)	6.	b)
2.	b)	7.	c)
3.	b)	8.	a)
4.	a)	9.	b)
5.	c)	10.	c)

Chapter 6

1.	a)	6.	a)
2.	b)	7.	b)
3.	a)	8.	b)
4.	c)	9.	c)
5.	c)	10.	a)

Chapter 7

1.	b)	6.	a)
2.	b)	7.	c)
3.	a)	8.	c)
4.	c)	9.	b)
5.	c)	10.	a)

Chapter 8

1.	b)	6.	b)
2.	a)	7.	a)
3.	c)	8.	b)
4.	b)	9.	b)
5.	c)	10.	c)

Chapter 9

1.	a)	6.	a)
2.	a)	7.	c)
3.	b)	8.	c)
4.	b)	9.	b)
5.	a)	10.	c)

Chapter 10

1.	c)	6.	c)
2.	a)	7.	b)
3.	c)	8.	a)
4.	b)	9.	b)
5.	a)	10.	b)

Chapter 11

1.	c)	6.	c)
2.	a)	7.	b)
3.	a)	8.	a)
4.	b)	9.	a)
5.	c)	10.	a)

Chapter 12

1.	c)	6.	a)
2.	b)	7.	a)
3.	a)	8.	b)
4.	b)	9.	a)
5.	b)	10.	c)

APPENDIX B

CROSSWORD PUZZLES _____

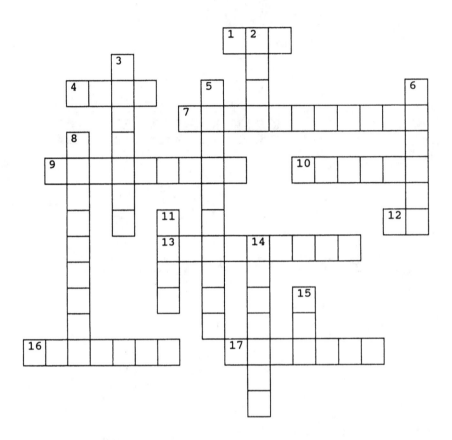

Puzzle #1 — Across

1. Recommended Dietary
   Allowances
4. Fluid produced by the liver and
   stored in the gallbladder
7. Chewing
9. Mottled enamel
10. Disease associated with a lack
    of vitamin C
12. Retinol Equivalent
13. Cracks along the edges of the lips
16. A deep crack or groove
17. Digestive enzyme found in the
    mouth

Puzzle #1 — Down

2. Food taken into the mouth
3. Blood sugar
5. Food which encourages dental
   decay
6. Causes a chemical change or
   break down in other substances
8. Inflammation of the tongue
11. Calorie
14. Anything that grows in a pea
    type of pod
15. High density lipoproteins

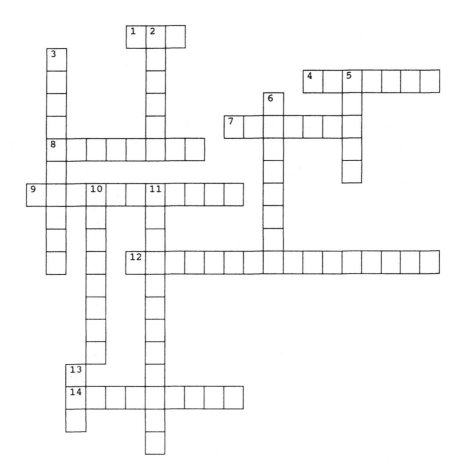

Puzzle #2 — Across

1. Parts per million
4. Table sugar
7. Excessive accumulation of body fat
8. A thiamin deficiency disorder
9. A mineral in solution that is able to conduct electric current
12. Loss of minerals in enamel due to acid attacks
14. The process by which foods are broken down into their nutrients

Puzzle #2 — Down

2. Bacteria and bacterial products that accumulate on teeth
3. The breaking down of body tissue
5. Semifluid mass food is converted into during digestion in stomach
6. A niacin deficiency disorder
10. Protein substance that holds body cells together
11. Abnormal thinning of bones in the elderly
13. Low density lipoproteins

Puzzle #1 Answer Key

```
                                    R  D  A
               G                       I
       B  I  L  E           C          E                    E
               U        M  A  S  T  I  C  A  T  I  O  N     N
       G       C           R                               Z
    F  L  U  O  R  O  S  I  S        S  C  U  R  V  Y       Y
       O       S           O                               M
       S       E     K     G                      R  E
       S             C  H  E  I  L  O  S  I  S
       I             A     N        E
       T             L     I        G        H
       I                   C        U        D
    F  I  S  S  U  R  E           A  M  Y  L  A  S  E
                                    E
                                    S
```

Across: RDA · BILE · MASTICATION · FLUOROSIS · SCURVY · CHEILOSIS · FISSURE · AMYLASE

Down: DIET · GLUCOSE · CARIOGENIC · ENZYME · GLOSSITIS · KCAL · LEGUMES · HDL

Puzzle #2   Answer Key

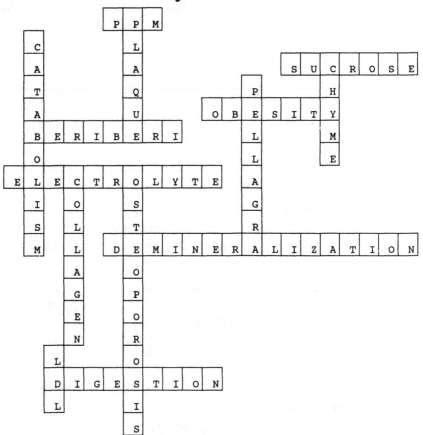

GLOSSARY

Absorption

The process of taking nutrients into the circulation system so that they can be used by the body.

Acid attack

The attack on dental enamel caused by the bacteria in plaque which occurs each time cariogenic foods are eaten.

Acidosis

A disorder characterized by an abnormally high level of acid in the blood or by a decrease in the alkali reserve in the body.

Amenorrhea

Lack of menstruation.

Amino acid

The fundamental structural units of proteins.

Amino acid, essential

An amino acid that cannot be synthesized rapidly enough by the body to meet the demands for normal health and growth.

Amino acid, nonessential

An amino acid that can be synthesized by the body in adequate quantities.

Amylase

The enzyme found in pancreatic juice that acts on starch.

Anabolism

The conversion of simple compounds derived from nutrients into substances that the body cells can use.

Anaerobic organisms

Bacteria that thrive only in the absence of oxygen.

Anemia

Reduction in the size or number of red blood cells, the quantity of hemoglobin, or both.

Anencephaly

A fatal birth defect in which part of the brain never develops. A lack of folic acid during early pregnancy may be a contributing factor.

Anorexia nervosa

An illness characterized by excessive, self-imposed weight loss and a distorted attitude toward eating and body weight.

Anti-cariogenic

Foods that inhibit dental decay.

Antioxidant

A substance that slows the deterioration of materials through the oxidation process.

Arachidonic acid

An essential fatty acid needed for normal growth, healthy skin, and reducing blood cholesterol.

Ariboflavinosis

A riboflavin deficiency disorder.

Ascorbic acid

Another name for vitamin C.

Aspartame

A nonnutritive sweetener.

BBS

Baby bottle syndrome characterized by a distinct pattern of rapid tooth decay in young children.

Basal metabolism

The least amount of energy needed to maintain essential life processes such as breathing, beating of the heart, circulation, and maintaining body temperature.

Beriberi

A thiamin deficiency disorder which, in its severe forms, affects the cardiovascular, muscular, and nervous systems.

Beta carotene

A precursor of vitamin A.

Bile

Fluid produced by the liver and stored in the gallbladder.

Binge eating

The rapid consumption of large amounts of food in a short period of time.

Biting

The use of the anterior teeth to cut or tear food into bite-size pieces.

Blood sugar

See **Glucose.**

Brown sugar

Sucrose crystals colored with molasses syrup.

Bulimia nervosa

A disorder characterized by recurrent episodes of binge eating followed by purging to get rid of the food which was eaten.

Calculus

Hardened deposits of dental plaque. Also known as tartar.

Calorie

The amount of heat required to raise the temperature of one gram of water by one degree Celsius.

Carbohydrates
Provide energy necessary to support life and come primarily from plant sources.

Cariogenic foods
Foods that can be utilized by dental plaque.

Canostatic
Foods that inhibit decay.

Catabolism
The breaking down of body tissues.

Cellulose
A form of dietary fiber that cannot be digested by humans.

Cheilosis
Cracks and fissures along the edges of the lips and at the corners of the mouth.

Chemical digestion
The action of enzymes as they break foods into simpler forms which can be absorbed by the body.

Chewing
The use of the posterior teeth to grind food before it is swallowed.

Cholesterol
A complex, fat-related compound found in practically all body tissues.

Chyme
Thick, semifluid mass into which food is converted during digestion in the stomach. The form of food as it passes from the stomach into the small intestine.

Clear liquid diet
Broths, gelatin, and clear liquids that are digested easily. Not generally required for dental patients.

Cobalamin
Another name for vitamin B_{12}.

Coenzyme
A substance that works in cooperation with enzymes. Coenzymes usually contain vitamins as part of their structure.

Collagen
A protein substance that holds body cells together.

Complementary proteins
Incomplete proteins from different sources that work together to supply missing or inadequate amino acids.

Complex carbohydrates
Naturally occurring sugars, mainly from plants.

Confectioner's sugar
Powdered sugar.

Constipation
The infrequent or difficult evacuation of feces.

Corn sugar
Made from cornstarch.

Corn sweetener
Liquid sugar made from the breakdown of cornstarch.

Corn syrup
Syrup made by the partial breakdown of cornstarch.

Cretinism
Stunted body growth and mental development as a result of inadequate maternal iodine intake during pregnancy.

Cyclamates
Nonnutritive sweeteners.

Decay
Dental caries or the destruction of tooth structure by repeated acid attacks on the enamel caused by plaque.

Dehydration

The loss of water from the body.

Demineralization

The beginning stages of dental decay in which minerals are lost from the enamel.

Dentifrices

Toothpastes.

Dextrose

See **Glucose.**

Diastolic pressure

One of the two measurements in blood pressure readings. It occurs when the heart ventricles relax. See **Systolic pressure.**

Diet

The food that is taken into the mouth.

Diet, adequate

A diet that meets all of the nutritional needs of an individual and provides some degree of protection for periods of increased needs.

Dietary fiber

That part of whole grains, vegetables, fruits, and nuts that resists digestion in the gastrointestinal tract.

Dietary fluorides

See **Fluorides, systemic.**

Dietary Guidelines for Americans

Issued by the U.S. Dept. of Agriculture (USDA) and the Dept. of Health and Human Services (HHS), these guidelines explain how to make healthier dietary and lifestyle choices.

Digestion

The process by which foods are broken down into their nutrients.

Disaccharides
Double sugars which must be broken down into a simpler form before they can be used by the body.

Diuretic
A substance that causes water to be excreted by the kidneys.

Dynamic equilibrium
See **Homeostasis.**

Electrolyte
A mineral which, when dissolved in solution, is capable of conducting an electric current.

Empty calories
Foods that provide only energy and no other nutrients.

Emulsification
The process of breaking down fats into smaller particles.

Energy
See **Calorie.**

Enzyme
A substance that causes a chemical change or breakdown in other substances.

ESIs
Estimated Safe and Adequate Daily Dietary Intakes. A form of measurement sometimes used when RDAs have not been established for a nutrient.

Estrogen replacement therapy
The artificial replacement of estrogen after menopause.

Facultative organisms
Bacteria that can thrive either in the presence or absence of oxygen.

Fats, monounsaturated
Fats from vegetable sources that neither raise nor lower the serum cholesterol level.

Fats, polyunsaturated
Fats from vegetable sources that tend to lower the serum cholesterol level.

Fats, saturated
Fats from animal sources that increase the serum cholesterol level.

Fat-soluble vitamins
Vitamins A, D, E, and K. They are stored in body fat.

Fats, unsaturated
Divided into two categories: monounsaturated and polyunsaturated. These fats generally have a neutral or slightly beneficial effect on blood cholesterol.

Fatty acids
A component of dietary fat. They come in two types: saturated and unsaturated.

Fatty acids, essential
Polyunsaturated fatty acids required by the body.

Feces
Solid wastes eliminated from the body through the rectum.

Fermentable carbohydrates
Complex carbohydrates that stay in the mouth long enough to be broken down into sugars by the action of salivary amylase.

Fissure
A deep groove.

Fluoride
An essential mineral that is known to strengthen teeth and bones and make teeth more resistant to acid attacks that cause dental decay.

Fluorides, systemic
Fluorides which are ingested in water, food, beverages, or supplements. Also known as dietary fluorides.

Fluorides, topical

Those fluorides which are applied in direct contact with the teeth through mouth rinses, fluoridated tooth paste, and topical fluoride applications. Also known as non-dietary fluorides.

Fluorosis, dental

Discoloration and weakening of enamel as the result of excessive fluoride intake. Also known as mottled enamel.

Folacin

Another name for folic acid.

Folate

Another name for folic acid.

Food Guide Pyramid

Introduced in 1992, this is the visual companion to the written Dietary Guidelines for Americans. It emphasizes eating a variety of foods in relative proportions. See **Dietary Guidelines for Americans.**

Fortified

Enrich or strengthen by adding ingredients such as vitamins A and D to whole milk.

Fructose

The monosaccharide found in ripe fruit, juices, and honey. Also known as fruit sugar and levulose.

Fruit juice concentrate

Used as the sweetener in many foods that are labeled "no sugar added."

Fruit sugar

See **Fructose.**

Full liquid diet

Foods that are liquid at room temperature or that liquify at body temperature.

Galactose

A monosaccharide which the liver converts into glucose.

Gastric juice

The liquid responsible for digestion in the stomach.

Glossitis

Inflammation of the tongue.

Glucose

The form of simple sugar found in some foods. Also known as dextrose. The form of sugar that is found in the blood. Also known as blood sugar.

Glycogen

The equivalent of starch but from animal sources. Also the form in which the body stores energy in the liver and muscles.

Goiter (Simple)

Enlargement of the thyroid gland due to a lack of iodine.

Gum

A form of dietary fiber.

HDL

High-density lipoprotein. Also known as good cholesterol because it helps to eliminate plaque build-up.

Health

A state of complete physical, mental, and social well-being and not merely the absence of disease or infirmity.

Hemicellulose

A form of dietary fiber.

Hemoglobin

The iron-containing portion of the red blood cells.

Homeostasis

The ability of the body to maintain the balance of its internal environment.

Honey
Produced by bees it contains slightly more fructose than glucose.

Hydrochloric acid
The primary ingredient of gastric juices.

Hydrogenation
The process whereby oils are changed into solid fats at room temperature.

Hypertension
High blood pressure.

Hypocalcemia
Abnormally low levels of calcium in the blood.

Ingested
Eaten or taken into the body.

Inorganic
Composed of matter other than plant or animal origin.

Insalivation
The process of mixing food with saliva.

International unit
IU, unit of measurement of some vitamins. Five international units equal one retinol equivalent.

Intestinal juice
A straw-colored alkaline fluid secreted by the intestinal mucosa. Intestinal juice contains enzymes that complete the hydrolysis of carbohydrates, protein, and fat.

Invert sugar
A mixture of glucose and fructose.

Kcal
See **Kilocalorie.**

Ketosis
A condition that is characterized by a sweetish acetone odor of the breath.

Key nutrients

Those that play the most important role: carbohydrates, proteins, fats, water, vitamins, and minerals.

Kilocalorie

1,000 times larger than a calorie.

Kwashiorkor

A nutritional deficiency disease caused by an inadequate intake of protein.

Lactase

The enzyme found in intestinal juice that works on lactose.

Lactose

A disaccharide found in milk. Also known as milk sugar.

LDL

Low-density lipoprotein, also known as bad cholesterol because it leads to plaque build-up.

Legumes

Anything that grows in a pea-type of pod. Legumes include peas, beans, lentils, and peanuts.

Levulose

See **Fructose.**

Lignin

A form of dietary fiber.

Linoleic acid

An essential fatty acid needed for normal growth, healthy skin, and reducing blood cholesterol.

Lipase

The enzyme found in gastric juice and pancreatic juice that works on emulsified fats.

Liquid formula foods

Commercially available preparations that include all necessary nutrients in varying caloric amounts.

Malnutrition

Any disorder of nutrition or undesirable health status that is due to either a lack of or an excess of nutrient supply.

Maltase

The enzyme found in intestinal juice that works on maltose.

Maltose

A disaccharide formed from the breakdown of starch in the small intestine.

Mannitol

A sugar alcohol.

Maple syrup

Made from the sap of the sugar maple tree.

Mastication

Chewing.

Mechanical digestion

The process of breaking food into smaller portions and mixing it with digestive juices.

Megadose

Ten times the RDA for water-soluble vitamins and five times the RDA for fat-soluble vitamins.

Metabolic rate

The speed and efficiency with which the body converts food into useful nutrients.

Metabolism

All of the chemical changes that determine the body's final use of nutrients.

Metabolism, basal

The least amount of energy needed to maintain essential life processes.

Microgram

One millionth of a gram (mcg).

Micromineral
See **Trace element.**

Milk sugar
See **Lactose.**

Milligram
One thousandth of a gram (mg).

Minerals
Inorganic substances that are necessary in minute amounts for proper growth, development, and optimal health.

Molasses
The syrup that is separated from raw sugar during processing.

Monosaccharides
Single sugars, the simplest form of carbohydrate.

Mottled enamel
See **Fluorosis.**

Niacinamide
Another name for niacin.

Nicotinic acid
Another name for niacin.

Night blindness
Changes in the eye that occur as the result of a vitamin A deficiency and cause defective or reduced vision in the dark.

Noncariogenic
Those foods which do not promote dental decay.

Nondietary fluorides
See **Fluorides, topical.**

Nonessential amino acids
Amino acids that can be synthesized by the body in adequate quantities to meet metabolic needs.

Nonnutritive sweeteners
Sweetening agents that do not contribute nutrients or significant calories to the diet.

Nutrient
Any chemical substance needed by the body for one or more of the following functions: to provide heat or energy, to build and repair tissues, and to regulate life processes.

Nutrient density
The amount of nutritional value received per calorie.

Nutrition
The manner in which the body utilizes the nutrients contained in foods which are eaten.

Nutrition, good
The body is well nourished by having received and put to work foods containing essential nutrients in the amounts needed.

Nutrition Labeling and Education Act (NLEA)
This law makes nutritional labeling mandatory for most foods.

Obesity
An accumulation of excessive fat in the body which results in body weight beyond the limitations of skeletal and physical requirements.

Organic
Composed of matter of plant or animal origin.

Osteomalacia
Abnormal softening of the bones.

Osteoporosis
A condition, usually occurring in the elderly, in which there is an excessive loss of bone mass or density that results in weakening and brittleness of the bones.

Overnutrition

The intake of excessive nutrients which may lead to obesity and its many related diseases.

Pancreatic juice

Digestive juice produced by the pancreas and secreted into the small intestine.

Pectin

A form of dietary fiber.

Pellagra

A niacin deficiency disorder which may result in death.

Pentosan

A form of dietary fiber.

Pepsin

The enzyme found in gastric juice that works on proteins.

Peptidase

The enzyme in intestinal juice that causes the breakdown of proteins and polypeptides into amino acids.

Peristalsis

A series of wave-like contractions that move food through the intestines.

Pernicious anemia

A form of anemia caused by a vitamin B_{12} deficiency.

Pit

The point at which two grooves cross on the chewing surface of a tooth.

Plaque, dental

Soft deposits that accumulate on the teeth and consist chiefly of bacteria and bacterial products.

Polysaccharides

Complex carbohydrates.

PPM

Parts per million.

Precursor

A substance from which another substance is formed.

Preformed vitamin A

Vitamin A from food sources such as liver, fish liver oils, eggs, and fortified whole milk.

Prophylaxis, dental

Professional cleaning of the teeth by the dentist or hygienist to remove plaque, calculus, and stains.

Protein-calorie nutrition
See **Kwashiorkor.**

Protein, complete

A food protein that contains all of the essential amino acids in significant amounts and in proportions fairly similar to those found in body protein.

Protein, incomplete

A food protein lacking one or more of the essential amino acids or supplying too little of an essential amino acid to support health.

PUFA

Polyunsaturated fatty acids.

Pyridoxal

Another name for vitamin B_6.

Pyridoxamine

Another name for vitamin B_6.

Pyridoxine

Another name for vitamin B_6.

Raw sugar

An intermediate product in the refining process, prohibited in the United States because of its impurities.

RDAs

Recommended Dietary Allowances. Recommendations for the average daily amounts of nutrients that population groups based on age and sex should consume over a period of time.

RDI

Reference Daily Intake. A new value used to replace the current U.S. RDAs.

Red disclosing tablet

A tablet consisting of a harmless red dye that is used to make plaque visible to the patient.

Remineralization

The process whereby demineralized enamel is repaired by the body.

Remodeling

A continuous maintenance or repair process resulting from the resorption of existing bone and the deposition of new bone to replace that which was removed.

Rennin

The enzyme found in gastric juice that works on milk proteins.

Retentiveness

Oral clearance time. How long it takes food to leave the mouth.

Retinol

Another name for vitamin A.

Retinol equivalent

RE, a unit of measurement of vitamin A.

Rickets

A condition in which there is a disturbance in the normal ossification (hardening) of the bones that is associated with a vitamin D deficiency.

Saccharin

A nonnutritive sweetener.

Salivary amylase
> The enzyme found in saliva that acts on carbohydrates.

Scurvy
> A disorder resulting from a severe deficiency of vitamin C.

Sealant
> A preventive dentistry measure to stop decay on the occlusal surfaces before it begins.

Serum cholesterol
> The amount of cholesterol circulating in the blood.

Simple carbohydrates
> Refined sugars, sweeteners added to processed foods, and natural sugar in honey and fruit.

Sorbitol
> A sugar alcohol.

Spina bifida
> A birth defect in which the spinal cord is not properly encased in bone. This may be caused by a lack of folate early in the pregnancy.

Starch
> A polysaccharide from plant sources.

Sucrase
> The enzyme found in intestinal juice that works on sucrose.

Sucrose
> A disaccharide that is a combination of glucose and fructose. Also known as table sugar.

Systolic pressure
> One of the two measurements in blood pressure readings. It occurs when the ventricles of the heart contract and push the blood out from the heart. See **Diastolic pressure.**

Table sugar
See **Sucrose.**

Tartar
See **Calculus.**

Total invert sugar
See **Invert sugar.**

Toxic
Poisonous.

Trace element
Minerals needed by the body in very small amounts.

Trans-fatty acid
The change that occurs in the unsaturated fatty acid chain when the oil is hydrogenated.

Trauma
Injury or wound.

Triglycerides
Complex molecules that comprise about 95 percent of dietary fat.

Trypsin
The enzyme found in pancreatic juice that acts on protein.

Turbinado
Partially refined sugar.

Undernutrition
An undesirable health status resulting from a lack of healthy nutrients. In the young it may inhibit growth, delay maturation, limit physical activity, and interfere with learning.

US RDAs
United States Recommended Daily Allowances.

Vitamins

Organic substances that are present in food in minute quantities and that perform specific functions for normal nutrition.

Water-soluble vitamins

Vitamins not stored in the body. An adequate supply of these vitamins must be consumed daily. They include vitamin C and the B-complex vitamins.

White spot lesion

Discoloration of the enamel which indicates the beginning of dental decay.

Xylitol

A sugar alcohol.

REFERENCES ──────────

"A Guide to Dental Care." *Consumer Reports* 57, no. 9 (September 1992): 601–16.

"An Eating Plan for Healthy Americans." *American Heart Association* (1991).

"Are You Eating Right?" *Consumer Reports* 57, no. 10 (October 1992): 644–55.

Banting, D. W. "The Future of Fluoride." *JADA* 123 (August 1991): 86–91.

Barbakow, F., et al. "Enamel Remineralizations: How to Explain it to Patients." *Quintessence-International* 22, no. 5 (May 1991): 341–47.

Baskin, Rosemary. "How Many Calories? How Much Fat?" *Consumer Reports Books.* Yonkers, NY: 1991.

Blumberg, J. B. "Dietary Antioxidants and Aging." *Contemporary Nutrition* 17, no. 3 (1992).

Brody, J. *Jane Brody's Good Food Book.* New York: Bantam Books, 1987.

Brody, J. *Jane Brody's Nutrition Book.* New York: Bantam Books, 1987.

Cariostatic Mechanisms of Fluoride. Princeton: Dental Resource Center, 1990.

Dennion, L. J., Bierman, E. L. Ferguson, J. M. *Straight Talk About Weight Control.* Mount Vernon: Consumers Union, 1991.

Diet and Caries. Princeton, NJ: Dental Resource Center, 1990.

Dietary Guidelines for Americans. 3rd ed. U.S. Dept. of Agriculture, U.S. Dept. of Health and Human Services, 1990.

Dunkin, A. "Cholesterol Management for All Seasons." *Business Week* (December 23, 1991): 96–97.

Dunkin, A. "Hypertension: Take Heart." *Business Week* (July 6, 1992): 84–85.

Dunne, L. J. *Nutrition Almanac.* 3rd ed. New York: McGraw-Hill Publishing Co., 1990.

"Eating and Aging." *Nutrition Letter* III, no. 13: 11.

"Eating Right." *Mayo Clinic Health Letter* 10, no. 10 (October 1992): 7.

"Fluoridated Fruit." *CDA* 20, no. 6 (June 1992): 18.

Fluoride Products—An Update For the 1990's. Princeton, NJ: Dental Resource Center, 1990.

Grembowski, D., et al. "How Fluoridation Affects Adult Dental Caries." *JADA* 123 (February 1992): 49–54.

Hermann, M. "New Label Laws." *American Health* XI, no. 1 (January/February 1992): 96.

Holli, B. B., Calabrese, R. J. *Communication and Education Skills: The Dietician's Guide.* 2nd ed. Philadelphia: Lea and Febiger, 1991.

How To Brush and Floss. Chicago: The American Academy of Periodontology, 1989.

"How to Lower Blood Pressure." *Consumer Reports* 57, no. 5 (May 1992): 300–02.

Jacob, J. A. "New Technology can Remineralize Teeth." *ADA News* 23, no. 18 (October 5, 1992): 27.

Jarvis, C. *Physical Examination and Health Assessment.* Philadelphia: W. B. Saunders Company, 1992.

Kraus, B. *The Dictionary of Sodium, Fats, and Cholesterol.* 2nd ed. New York: Perigee Books, 1990.

"Living Alone: Can Social Isolation Affect your Health?" *Mayo Clinic Health Letter* 10, no. 9 (September 1992): 4–5.

Long, P. "It's Lunchtime: Do You Know What Your Kid's Cholesterol Is?" *Eating Well* 3, no. 14 (November/December 1992): 45–49.

Lucas, A. R. "Update and Review of Anorexia Nervosa." *Contemporary Nutrition* 14, no. 9 (1989).

Mason, J. O. "Too Much of a Good Thing?" *JADA* 122 (August 1991): 93–96.

Matschek, C. "What Message are You Sending?" *Dental Economics* 82, no. 11 (November 1992): 63–73.

Mitchel, J. E. "Bulimia Nervosa." *Contemporary Nutrition* 14, no. 10 (1989).

Murray, J. J., Rugg-Gunn, A. J., Jenkins, G. N. *Fluorides in Caries Prevention.* Oxford: Wright, 1991.

"New Advice for 70 Million Americans." *University of California At Berkeley Wellness Letter* 9, no. 2 (November 1992): 1–2.

Newbrun, E. "Preventing Dental Caries: Breaking the Chain of Transmission." *JADA* 123 (June 1992): 55–59.

Newbrun, E. "Preventing Dental Caries: Current and Prospective Strategies." *JADA* 123 (May 1992): 68–73.

Nizel, A. E., Papas, E. S. *Nutrition in Clinical Dentistry.* 3rd ed. Philadelphia: W. B. Saunders Company, 1989.

Palmer, C. "Water Fluoridation Still a Great Deal." *ADA News* (July 13, 1992): 13.

Pennington, J. A. *Bowes and Church's Food Values of Portions Commonly Used.* 15th ed. New York: Harper and Row, 1989.

Pradad, A. S., et al. "Role of Zinc in Human Nutrition." *Contemporary Nutrition* 16, no. 5 (1991).

Recommended Dietary Allowances. 10th ed. Washington, D.C.: National Academy Press, 1989.

Snow-Harter, C. "Exercise, Calcium and Estrogen: Primary Regulators of Bone Mass." *Contemporary Nutrition* 17, no. 4 (1992).

Stipp, D. "Heart-Attack Study Adds to the Cautions About Iron in the Diet." *The Wall Street Journal* (September 8, 1992): A1 and A5.

Stipp, D. "Warnings About Ingesting Too Much Iron." *The Wall Street Journal* (January 17, 1992): B1 and B3.

Tanouye, E. "Study Says Estrogen Treatments Reduce Fractures in Women With Osteoporosis." *The Wall Street Journal* (July 1, 1992): B6.

"The Anti-Cancer B Vitamin." *University of California at Berkeley Wellness Letter* 8, no. 13 (September 1991): 1.

"The Trouble with Margarine." *Consumer Reports* 56, no. 3 (March 1991): 196–97.

Toufexis, A. "The New Scoop on Vitamins." *Time*, April 6, 1992): 54–59.

Tribole, E. *Eat Right America: Your Guide to Achieving a Lowfat Lifestyle.* The American Dietetic Association, March 1992.

Tylenda, C. A., et al. "Bulimia Nervosa: Its Effect On Salivary Chemistry." *JADA* 122 (June 1991): 37–41.

USDA's Food Guide Pyramid. U.S. Dept. of Agriculture Home and Garden, Bulletin Number 249.

Woteki, C. E. "Nutrition in Childhood and Adolescence, Part I." *Contemporary Nutrition* 17, no. 1 (1992).

Woteki, C. E. "Nutrition in Childhood and Adolescence, Part II." *Contemporary Nutrition* 17, no. 2 (1992).

INDEX

Absorption, 20–21
  defined, 12
Acidosis, defined, 41
Acid attacks, 3, 184
Acids, essential fatty (EFAs),
  66
Acute necrotizing ulcerative
  gingivitis (ANU6), 162
Adolescence, nutritional
  needs of, 137
Adults
  nutritional needs of, 140
  wound healing and, 153–54
Alveolar bone loss, 146–47
Amenorrhea, 62, 138
Amino acids, 59–60
Amylase, defined, 19
Anabolism, 21–22
Anacephaly, 84
Anemia, 98
Anorexia nervosa, 138
Anticariogenic foods, 184
Antimicrobial rinses, 198
Antioxidants, 72
Arachidonic, 66
Ariboflavinosis, 82
Ascorbic acid, 78–79
Aspartame, 49

Baby-bottle syndrome (BBS),
  134

Basal metabolism rate, 34
BBS. *See* Baby-bottle
  syndrome.
Beans, eggs, and nuts food
  group, 118, 121
B-complex deficiency, 80–81
  cheilosis, 80
  glossitis, 80
Beriberi, 81
Beta carotene, 73
Bile, defined, 18
Binge eating, 138
Biotin, 85
Blood pressure, readings,
  142–43
Blood sugar, 43, 45, 46
Bone formation, 140
Bread, cereal, rice, and
  pasta food group, 120,
  121
Brown sugar, 46
Bulimia nervosa, 138–40
  dental implications,
  139–40

Calcium, 93–95, 147–48
  absorption and, 95
  content of in popular
  foods, 94
  supplements, 95
Calcium carbonate, 95

Calculus, 183
Calories
    daily requirements, 35
    defined, 34
    empty, 36
    per nutrient, 35, 36
Carbohydrates, 40–56
    cariogenicity of, 184–86
    classifications of, 42–45
    complex, 42
    defined, 27
    fermentable, 185
    functions of, 41
    information about on food
        labels, 123
    refined, 42
    simple, 185
    sources of, 42
Cariogenic, defined, 184
Catabolism, 21
Cellulose, 44, 45, 49
Cheilosis, 80
Children
    preschool, nutritional
        needs of, 135
    school-age, 136
Chloride, 107
Cholesterol, 141
Chromium, 103–4
Chyme, defined, 17
Clear liquid diet, 155
Cobalamin, 84
Coenzymes, defined, 14
Collagen, 78
Complementary proteins, 62
Complete protein, 61
Confectioner's sugar, 46
Constipation, defined, 20

Copper, 101
Corn sugar, 46
Corn sweetner, 46
Corn syrup, 47
Cretinism, 100
Cyclamates, 49

Decay. See Dental caries.
Dehydration, 67
Demineralization, 170–71
Dental caries, 185–87
    major dietary factors in,
        186
Dental decay, causes of, 3
Dental fluorosis, 169
Dental patients
    diets for, 153–64
    acute necrotizing ulcera-
        tive gingivitis (ANU6),
        162
    immediate denture, 164
    liquid, 155, 156
    modified and special
        needs, 158–63
    new dentures, 163–64
    oral surgery, 163
    orthodontic patients,
        160–61
    periodontal surgery,
        162–63
    soft, 155, 157
    supplementation of, 158
    temporomandibular joint
        (TMJ) problems, 160
    wired jaws, 159
    wound healing, 153–54
Dental prophylaxis, defined,
    183

Dentistry
diet and preventive, 2–3
role of sealants in, 135
fluorides and, 168–73
Dentition, effects of loss of,
144
Dentrifices, 189–90
Dentures, diet and, 163–64
Dextrose, 43, 46
Diet
adequate, defined, 5
guidelines for maintaining
healthy weight, 113–17
Diet diary, 125–26
form, 126
Dietary fats, 63
Dietary fiber, 49–53
content of in popular
foods, 52
functions of, 50
insoluble, 51
requirements of, 51–53
soluble, 50–51
sources of, 50–51
Dietary Guidelines for Americans, 112
Digestion, 12–20
absorption and, 20–21
changes in the mouth,
16–17
chemical reactions in, 15
defined, 12
large intestine and, 19–20
mechanical and chemical,
12, 17–19
small intestine and, 18–19
stomach, 17–18
Digestive action, sites of, 14

Digestive system, major
structures of, 13
Disaccharides, 44
Disclosing agents, 188
Diuretic, 67, 105
Dynamic equilibrium,
defined, 21

Eating, frequency of, 189–90
EFA. See Essential fatty acids
Elderly
effects of lost dentition, 144
nutritional needs of, 143
Electrolytes, 105–7
Elimination, defined, 20
Empty calories, 36
Emulsification, 18
Enzymes, defined, 12, 15
Essential amino acids
(EFAs), 66
Estimated safe and adequate
daily dietary intakes
(ESIs), 30, 73
Estrogen replacement ther-
apy osteoporosis and, 148
Exercise, osteoporosis and,
147

Fat
information about on food
labels, 123
percentage in food, calcu-
lation, 115–16
Fats, 62–66
cholesterol, 141
content of in popular
foods, 61
defined, 27

dietary, 63
function of, 62
oils, content of, 65
polyunsaturated (PUFA), 65
saturated, 63–64
sources of, 63
unsaturated, 63, 65
Fatty acids, 63
Fiber, dietary, 49–53
content of in popular
    foods, 52
functions of, 50
insoluble, 51
requirements of, 51–53
soluble, 50–51
sources of, 50–51
Flossing, technique, 194–97
Fluoridated water, 172–73
Fluoride, supplements
during prenatal develop-
    ment, 170
infancy, 173–74
birth to 3 years, 170
adult, 170
for high-risk patients,
    171–72
in water, 172–73
prescribed, 173
Fluorides, 3, 102–3. 168–73
dietary, 168
nondietary, 169
systemic, 168, 171–72
topical, 168–69, 175–77
Folacin, 84
Folate, 84
Folic acid, 84
Food
cariogenic, 185

physical characteristics of,
    184
retentiveness, 187
plaque and, 182–84
Food groups, 118–22
beans, eggs, and nuts,
    118, 121
bread, cereal, rice, and
    pasta, 120–21
meat, poultry, and fish,
    118, 120
milk, yogurt, and cheese,
    118, 120
nonessential, 118, 121
vegetable and fruit, 118,
    120
Food Guide Pyramid, 117–22
Food labeling, 123
nutrition information on,
    123–24
carbohydrate information,
    123–24
fat information, 123–24
information per serving,
    123–24
percentage of U.S. RDA,
    124
sodium and, 123–24
Fructose, 43, 47
Fruit juice concentrate, 47
Fruit sugar, 43
Full liquid diet, 155, 156

Galactose, 43, 44
Gastric juice, defined, 17
Glossitis, 80
Glucose, 43, 45, 46
Glycogen, 44, 45

Goiter, 99
Gum, 49

Health, defined, 7
Hemicellulose, 49
High blood pressure, 142
    classification of, 143
Homeostasis, defined, 21
Honey, 48
Hydrochloric acid, 17
Hydrogenated oils, 66
Hypertension, 142
    classification of, 143
Hypocalcemia, 76

Incomplete protein, 62
Infancy
    fluoride supplements dur-
        ing, 173
    nutritional needs during,
        133–34
Inorganic substances, de-
    fined, 28
Insalivation, defined, 16
Interproximal brushes, 198
Intestinal juice, defined, 19
Iodine, 99–100
Iron, 97–98
Iron deficiency anemia, 98

Ketosis, defined, 41
Kilocalorie, defined, 34
Kwashiorkor, 58

Lactase, defined, 19
Lactose, 44
Large intestine, digestion
    and, 19–20

Levulose, 43, 47
Lignin, 49
Linoleic acid, 66
Lipase, defined, 18, 19
Lipoproteins, 141–42
    high-density, 141–42
    low-density, 141–42
Lips, B-complex deficiency
    and, 80
Liquid diets, 155, 156

Magnesium, 96–97
Malnutrition, defined, 5
Maltase, defined, 19
Maltose, 44
Manganese, 102
Mannitol, 49
Maple syrup, 48
Mastication, 16
Maternal nutritional care,
    133
Meats, poultry, and fish food
    group, 118, 120
Megadose, defined, 31
Metabolism, 21–22
    basal, 34
    defined, 12, 21
Microminerals, 92
Milk, yogurt, and cheese
    food group, 118, 120
Milk sugar, 44
Minerals, 91–101
    absorption of, 95
    calcium, 93–95
    content of in popular
        foods, 94
    chloride, 107
    chromium, 103–4

classification of, 91–92
copper, 101
defined, 28
functions of, 91
iodine, 99–100
iron, 97–98
magnesium, 96–97
manganese, 102
molybdenum, 104
phosphorus, 95–96
potassium, 105
selenium, 100–1
sodium, 106
zinc, 98–99
Modified diets, 158–63
    acute necrotizing ulcerative
        gingivitis (ANUG) and,
        162
    dentures and, 163–64
    injured anterior teeth and,
        158–59
    oral surgery and, 163
    orthodontic appliances
        and, 160–61
    periodontal surgery and,
        162–63
    temporomandibular joint
        (TMJ) problems and, 160
    wired jaw and, 159
    wound healing and, 153–54
Molasses, 48
Molybdenum, 104
Monosaccharides, 43
Mottled enamel, 169
Mouthwashes, 198

Niacin, 82–83
Niacinamide, 82

Nicotinic acid, 82
Night blindness, 75
Nonessential amino acids,
    59–60
Nutrient density, 35–36
Nutrients
    defined, 27
    key, 27
    purpose of, 28–29
    Recommended Dietary Al-
        lowances (RDAs), 29–31
Nutrition
    defined, 5
    general, 2–3
    theories, 6–7
Nutrition Labeling and Edu-
    cation Act (NLEA), 123
Nutritional disorders
    anorexia nervosa, 138
    bulimia nervosa, 138–40
    high blood pressure, 142
    hypertension, 142
    obesity, 5
    oral manifestations of, 80
    anemia, 98
    ariboflavinosis, 82
    B-complex, 80–81
    pellagra, 82
    rickets, 76
    scurvy, 79
    osteoporosis, 146–48
Nutritional needs, 115–130
    adolescence, 137
    adulthood, 140
    effects of lost dentition, 144
    elderly, 143
    infancy, 133–34
    orthodontics, 160–61

prenatal and pregnancy,
132
preschool, 135
school-age children, 136
specialized, 145–46
wound healing, 153–54
Nutritional status
factors influencing, 143–44

Obesity, 5
Oral mucosa, B-complex deficiency and, 80
Organic substances, defined,
28
Orthodontic requirements,
modified diets and,
160–61
Orthodontics, nutritional
considerations in,
160–61
Osteomalacia, 76
Osteoporosis, 76, 140,
146–48
alveolar bone loss, 146–47
daily exercise and, 147
estrogen replacement therapy, 148
treatment and prevention
of, 147–48
Overnutrition, defined, 5

Pancreatic juice, defined, 19
Pantothenic acid, 86
Pectin, 49
Pellagra, 82
Pentosan, 49
Pepsin, defined, 17
Peptidases, defined, 19

Periodontal disease, plaque
and, 182–84
Periodontal surgery, diets
and, 162–63
Peristalsis, defined, 12, 41
Pernicious anemia, 85
Personal oral hygiene (POH),
187–88
Phosphorus, 95–96
Plaque
bacteria associated with,
182–83
defined, 182
diet, dental disease and, 4,
182–84
foods and, 184–88
removal of, 183
Polysaccharides, 44
Potassium, 105
Pregnancy, nutritional needs
during, 132
Prenatal
dental development, 132
nutritional needs, 132
Preschool child, nutritional
needs of, 135
Preventive dentistry. See
Dentistry, preventive
Protein-calorie malnutrition,
58
Proteins, 58–62
complete and incomplete,
61–62
content of in popular
foods, 61
defined, 27
functions of, 58
sources of, 59

Pyridoxal, 83
Pyridoxamine, 83
Puridoxine, 83

Recommended Dietary Allow-
    ances (RDAs), 29–31, 73
Reference Daily Intake (RDI),
    31
Remineralization, 170–71
Rennin, defined, 17
Rententiveness, 187
Retinol, 74
Riboflavin, 82
Rickets, 76

Saccharin, 49
Saliva, role in digestion,
    16–17
Salivary amylase, defined, 16
Saturated fats, 63–64
School-age child, nutritional
    needs of, 136
Scurvy, 79
Selenium, 100–1
Serum cholesterol, 141–42
Small intestine, digestion
    and, 18–19
Sodium, 106
    information about on food
        labels, 123–24
Soft diets, 155, 157
Sorbitol, 49
Spina bifida, 84
Starch, 44, 45
Stim-u-dents, 198
Stomach, digestion and,
    17–18
Sucrase, defined, 19

Sucrose, 44, 46
Sugar, 42–49
    cariogenicity of, 184
    content of in popular
        foods, 47
    information about on food
        labels, 123–24
    invert, 48
    raw, 48
Sugar alcohols, 49
Supplements
    calcium, 95
    fluoride, 173
    guidelines for taking, 31–33
    prescribed fluoride, 168–69
Sweetners
    nonnutritive, 49
    nutritive, 46–49

Table sugar, 44
Tartar, 183
Teeth
    injured anterior, 158–59
Teeth cleaning aids, 197–98
Temporomandibular joint
    (TMJ) problems,
    diet for, 160
Thiamin, 81
Tongue, B-complex defi-
    ciency and, 80–81
Toothbrush selection, 189
Toothbrushing technique,
    190–93
Toothpastes, 189–90
Total invert sugar, 48
Trace elements, 101–4
Trans-fatty acid, 66
Triglycerides, 63

Trypsin, defined, 19
Turbinado, 48

Undernutrition, defined, 5
United States Recommended
    Daily Allowances (U.S.
    RDAs), 31
    food labels and, 124
Unsaturated fats, 63, 65

Vegetable and fruit group,
    118, 120
Vitamin A, 74–75
Vitamin B complex,
    79–86
    Vitamin B1, 81
    Vitamin B2, 82
    Vitamin B3, 82–83
    Vitamin B6, 83
    Vitamin B12, 84–85
Vitamin C, 78–79
Vitamin D, 75–76
Vitamin E, 76–77
Vitamin K, 77–78
Vitamins, 72–86

daily needs, 73
defined, 28
fat soluble, 72, 74–77
functions of, 72
measurements, 73
water soluble, 72, 78–86

Water, 66–67
defined, 28
fluoridated, 173
functions of, 66–67
sources of, 67
Weight
control, 113
control and role of nutri-
    tion, 113, 116–17
suggested range for adults,
    chart, 114
Wired jaw, diet for, 159
Wound healing, nutritional
    needs during, 153–54

Xylitol, 49

Zinc, 98–99

CPSIA information can be obtained
at www.ICGtesting.com
Printed in the USA
FFHW010312061218
49770703-54244FF